中国罕见病
防治与保障事业发展
（第2版）

Prevention and Treatment of Rare Diseases in China
and the Development of Social Security System

（Second Edition）

国家卫生健康委员会　编

National Health Commission of the People's Republic of China

中国协和医科大学出版社

北　京

图书在版编目（CIP）数据

中国罕见病防治与保障事业发展 / 国家卫生健康委员会编. —2版. —北京：中国协和医科大学出版社，2024.1
ISBN 978-7-5679-2265-5

Ⅰ.①中…　Ⅱ.①国…　Ⅲ.①疑难病－防治－研究－中国　②疑难病－医疗保健事业－研究－中国　Ⅳ.①R442.9

中国国家版本馆CIP数据核字（2023）第189160号

中国罕见病防治与保障事业发展（第2版）

编　　　者：	国家卫生健康委员会
责任编辑：	李元君
封面设计：	邱晓俐
责任校对：	张　麓
责任印制：	张　岱

出版发行：中国协和医科大学出版社
（北京市东城区东单三条9号　邮编100730　电话010-65260431）

网　　址：	www.pumcp.com
经　　销：	新华书店总店北京发行所
印　　刷：	涿州汇美亿浓印刷有限公司

开　　本：	710mm×1000mm　　1/16
印　　张：	6.75
字　　数：	75千字
版　　次：	2024年1月第2版
印　　次：	2024年1月第1次印刷
定　　价：	35.00元

ISBN 978-7-5679-2265-5

编者名单

主　审　焦雅辉

主　编　张抒扬　李大川　李林康

副主编　张文宝　赵　琨　顾学范　邵　蓉
　　　　　　刘军帅　吴　晶

编　者（按姓氏笔画排序）

王　瑾　　王奕鸥　　王曼莉　　王耀羚

毛立坡　　田保国　　刘　鹏　　刘军帅

刘念启　　江虎军　　孙瑞娟　　李　娜

李大川　　李林康　　李剑思　　杨　胜

郝媛媛　　吴　晶　　张　楠　　张　蔚

张丁丁　　张文宝　　张西凡　　张抒扬

陈昌雄　　陈敬丹　　邵　蓉　　林荣杰

郑佳音　　赵　琨　　费珊龙　　顾学范

徐晓强　　高　颖　　唐旭东　　陶田甜

谢诗桐

Editor List

Reviewer

Jiao Yahui

Chief Editors

Zhang Shuyang, Li Dachuan, Li Linkang

Associate Editors

Zhang Wenbao, Zhao Kun, Gu Xuefan, Shao Rong,

Liu Junshuai, Wu Jing

Editors

Wang Jin, Wang Yiou, Wang Manli, Wang Yaoling, Mao Lipo,

Tian Baoguo, Liu Peng, Liu Junshuai, Liu Nianqi, Jiang Hujun,

Sun Ruijuan, Li Na, Li Dachuan, Li Linkang, Li Jiansi,

Yang Sheng, Bing Yuanyuan, Wu Jing, Zhang Nan,

Zhang Wei, Zhang Dingding, Zhang Wenbao, Zhang Xifan,

Zhang Shuyang, Chen Changxiong, Chen Jingdan, Shao Rong,

Lin Rongjie, Zheng Jiayin, Zhao Kun, Fei Shanlong,

Gu Xuefan, Xu Xiaoqiang, Gao Ying, Tang Xudong,

Tao Tiantian, Xie Shitong

前　言

中国共产党第十八次全国代表大会以来，以习近平同志为核心的党中央始终坚持把人民生命安全和身体健康放在第一位。习近平总书记作出"没有全民健康，就没有全面小康"的重要论断，要求完善国民健康政策，为人民群众提供全方位全周期健康服务，把"实施健康中国战略"提升到国家整体战略层面统筹谋划。国务院政府工作报告中多次提出，加强重大疾病防控，加强罕见病用药保障。中国共产党第二十次全国代表大会进一步明确了中国发展的战略目标，明确了健康中国建设的任务，罕见病这一特殊疾病领域越来越受到国家与社会各方的关注。

目前，全球已知的罕见病超过7000种，其中大多数威胁患者生命，给患者和社会带来了沉重的疾病与经济负担。近年来，我国政府对罕见病保障工作给予全方位支持，取得了巨大突破和进展。2020年，在国家卫生健康委员会指导下，由中国罕见病联盟组织罕见病诊疗、医疗保障和社会保障、医学遗传、卫生经济学、公共卫生、医学伦理等领域专家编写了《中国罕见病防治与保障事业发展》，书籍梳理了中国罕见病的预防诊疗、科学研究、药品供应保障、社会保障和国际合作工作，集中展现了中国政府高度重视并积极推进罕见病防治工作。经国家卫生健康委员会、科学技术部、工业和信息化部、民政部、财政部、人力资源和社会保障部、国家医疗保障局、国家药品监督管理局、国家中医药管理局、国家自然科学基金委员会共同审核，于 2021 年初正式出版。

两年来，随着我国社会各界对罕见病领域的重视不断加强，多项政策陆续出台，各项成果不断涌现。为了更好地梳理与更新我国在罕见病领域的工作进展，2023 年我们对《中国罕见病防治与保障事业发展》进行修订，形成第 2 版。在此，我们向所有参与编写和审核工作的专家、学者及参与单位表示由衷感谢！

在新时代中国人民对美好生活新追求的引领下，进一步健全罕见病防治与保障相关政策制度、提升罕见病临床诊治水平、加强罕见病药品供应保障、完善罕见病社会保障体系，对我国罕见病防治水平的提升、社会保障体系的完善以及"全民健康"目标的实现，具有十分重大的意义。

我们相信，在党和政府的坚强领导和全社会的关怀下，中国必将进一步提升罕见病防治水平、优化罕见病保障政策，形成中国特色方案，并在国际罕见病诊疗保障领域发出中国声音。

编　者

2023 年 8 月

Preface

Since the 18th National Congress of the Communist Party of China (CPC), the CPC Central Committee with Comrade Xi Jinping as its core has given top priority to people's safety and health. President Xi Jinping put forward an important instruction that "prosperity for all is impossible without health for all". He called for improvement in China's national health policy, comprehensive full-life cycle health services for the people, and prioritizing Healthy China Initiative as a national plan of the country. In the government work report, the State Council repeatedly requested that more efforts should be made to prevent and control major diseases and guarantee the supply of orphan drugs. The 20th National Congress of the Communist Party of China has further defined China's strategic development goals and the tasks to build a Healthy China. Rare disease, a special field of diseases, is receiving attention from all sides of the country and society.

At present, there are more than 7,000 known rare diseases worldwide, most of which threaten the lives of patients and impose a heavy economic burden on the society. In recent years, the Chinese government has provided all-round support for social security related to rare diseases and has made great breakthroughs and progresses. In

2020, the first edition of the *Prevention and Treatment of Rare Diseases in China and the Development of Social Security System* was edited by the National Health Commission. China Alliance for Rare Disease invites experts from multiple fields, such as diagnosis and treatment of rare diseases, healthcare security and social security, medical genetics, health economics, and public health, to form the editing committee. This book reviews China's efforts in coping with rare diseases, including prevention, diagnosis, treatment, scientific research, medicine supply, social security, and international cooperation, fully demonstrating the Chinese government's great importance and active promotion of the prevention, diagnosis and treatment of rare diseases. In early 2021, joint efforts from the National Health Commission, the Ministry of Science and Technology, the Ministry of Industry and Information Technology, the Ministry of Civil Affairs, the Ministry of Finance, the Ministry of Human Resources and Social Security, the National Healthcare Security Administration, the National Medical Products Administration, the National Administration of Traditional Chinese Medicine, and the National Natural Science Foundation of China, were made in revising and finalizing the first edition.

Over the past two years, with the increasing attention paid to the field of rare diseases across various sectors of society, a number of policies have been issued one after another, and numerous achievements have emerged. In order to review and update the progress in the field of rare diseases in China, the *Prevention and Treatment of Rare Diseases in China and the Development of Social Security System* (Second Edition) was developed in 2023. We hereby sincerely thank all experts, departments and participating organizations for drafting and revising this book!

To better meet the Chinese people's new pursuit of a better life in the new era, it is of great significance to further improve the policies and systems related to the prevention, treatment and support of rare diseases, enhance the level of clinical diagnosis and treatment of rare diseases, strengthen guarantee for the supply of orphan drugs, and improve the social security system for rare diseases so as to better prevent and treat rare diseases in our country, to improve the social security system and to achieve the goal of "Health for All."

We are confident that under the firm leadership of the Party and the Chinese government and with social care, China will further improve prevention and treatment of rare diseases, refine security policies of rare diseases, put forward a plan with Chinese characteristics, and make our voice heard in the international community for the diagnosis, treatment and support of rare diseases.

Editing Committee

August 2023

目　录

第一章　政府高度重视罕见病防治工作·······················1

第二章　切实加强罕见病预防与诊疗·····················6

一、预防为主，降低罕见病发生率 ··········6

（一）大力推进一级预防 ···············7

（二）不断强化二级预防 ···············8

（三）逐步落实三级预防 ···············9

二、分类施策，解决不同类别罕见病问题 ···········10

（一）对有治疗或干预手段的罕见病加强诊疗管理 ·······10

（二）对尚无治疗或干预手段的罕见病加强医学研究 ·····13

（三）多部门综合施策，稳步推进罕见病防治工作 ·····13

第三章　不断推进罕见病科学研究·················14

一、战略布局，逐步攻克罕见病重大科技难题 ········14

（一）科学技术部部署罕见病重点攻关项目 ········14

（二）新药专项布局罕见病药物研发攻关 ········15

（三）中医药布局罕见病防治攻关 ·········16

二、广泛覆盖，逐步开展罕见病相关自由探索研究 ·····17

第四章　持续提升罕见病药品供应保障水平················18

一、建立罕见病药品研发创新的法制化保障体系 ······18

二、国家财税政策支持罕见病药品研发和引进 ······19

三、审评审批制度改革助力罕见病药品快速上市 ………… 20

四、罕见病药物卫生技术评估助力罕见病药品可及 ………… 21

五、药品供应保障相关举措逐步推进罕见病用药可及 ……… 22

第五章　稳步建设罕见病保障体系……………………………… 25

一、罕见病医疗保障 ………………………………………… 25

（一）制度政策设置 ……………………………………… 25

（二）降低成本举措 ……………………………………… 27

（三）地方探索经验 ……………………………………… 27

二、罕见病社会保障 ………………………………………… 28

（一）加大社会救助力度 ………………………………… 28

（二）扩大社会保险覆盖范围 …………………………… 29

（三）调动社会力量参与 ………………………………… 30

（四）促进商业保险补充保障 …………………………… 30

第六章　积极参与罕见病防治国际合作…………………………… 32

结束语…………………………………………………………… 33

Contents

I . Government Attaches Great Importance to the
Prevention and Treatment of Rare Diseases ················· 34

II . Effective Improvement of the Prevention and
Treatment of Rare Diseases ································· 43

  1. "Prevention as priority" for reduced incidence of
rare diseases ··43

    (1) Great efforts have been devoted to primary prevention ······46

    (2) Continuous progresses have been recorded in
strengthening secondary prevention ····················47

    (3) Steady advancement has been achieved in improving
tertiary prevention ····································48

  2. Targeted measures for rare diseases of different
categories ··50

    (1) Strengthened diagnosis and treatment for rare diseases
with proven treatment or intervention measures ··············50

    (2) Strengthened medical research on rare diseases for
which there is no proven treatment or
intervention measures yet ····························56

(3) Inter-departmental coordinated mechanism yielded steady

outcomes in rare disease prevention and treatment··········56

Ⅲ. Continuous Advancement of Scientific Research on

Rare Diseases ·· 58

1. Overcome major scientific and technological problems of

rare diseases step by step through strategic layout ··············59

(1) The Ministry of Science and Technology deploys key

research projects ···59

(2) New drug special projects for rare disease research and

development ··61

(3) TCM supports research on the prevention and

treatment of rare diseases ··62

2. Extensive explorations and researches on rare diseases ·········63

Ⅳ. Continuous Improvement of Supply of Orphan Drugs ······· 64

1. Establishment of law-based guarantee framework for

R&D of orphan drugs ··64

2. National financial and tax policy for R&D and

introduction of orphan drugs···66

3. Reform of the review and approval system to

accelerate marketing of orphan drugs ····························67

4. Health technology assessment of orphan drugs help

improve accessibility of orphan drugs ····························70

5. Relevant measures ensuring drug supply for

better accessibility of orphan drugs ·······························71

Ⅴ. Steady Progress of the Social Security System for
    Rare Diseases ·· 76
    1. Medical insurance for rare diseases ····················76
       (1) Systems and policies ·····························76
       (2) Measures to reduce costs························80
       (3) Local pilots and experience····················80
    2. Social security for rare diseases ·····················81
       (1) Strengthened social assistance ················82
       (2) Expanded coverage of social insurance ········83
       (3) Encouraged social participation ···············84
       (4) Highlight the supplementary role of
           commercial insurance ·························85
Ⅵ. Active Participation in International Cooperation of
    Rare Diseases Prevention and Treatment ··············· 87
Conclusion··· 89

第一章　政府高度重视罕见病防治工作

"健康是促进人的全面发展的必然要求，是经济社会发展的基础条件，是民族昌盛和国家富强的重要标志，也是广大人民群众的共同追求。"在2016年全国卫生与健康大会上，习近平总书记的重要讲话深刻阐述了推进健康中国建设的重大意义，是指导新形势下我国卫生与健康事业发展的纲领性文件。中国共产党第二十次全国代表大会对新时代新征程推进健康中国建设作出新的战略部署、赋予新的任务使命，提出"把保障人民健康放在优先发展的战略位置，完善人民健康促进政策"。贯彻习近平总书记关于卫生与健康重要论述，必须提升对罕见病的诊疗能力、提高医疗卫生服务的公平性和质量水平。加强罕见病等重大疾病防治，事关亿万群众福祉。

罕见病是一类发病率、患病率极低的疾病的总称。全球已知罕见病达7000余种，且每年新发现的罕见病以250种至280种疾病数量增长。据估算，全球有2.63亿至4.46亿罕见病患者，其中我国约有2000万罕见病患者。全球有获批的相应治疗方案或药物的病种不到10%，且大多需终身药物治疗。

鉴于现阶段国情和罕见病管理水平，我国目前尚未对罕见病进行法律界定，而是以目录的方式加以管理。2018年5月，国家卫生健康委员会、科学技术部、工业和信息化部、国家药品监督管理局、国家中医药管理局五部门联合发布了我国《第一批罕见病目录》，收录了121种罕见病，首次以目录的形式"界定"了罕见病，具有里程碑式的意义。该目录由不同领域权威专家根据我国人口疾病罹患情况、医疗技术水平、疾病负担和保障水平等，参考国际经验遴选产生。未来，相关部门还将按照分批制订、动态更新的工作程序与目标，逐步完善我国罕见病目录，2023年9月18日，国家卫生健康委、科学技术部、工业和信息化部、国家药监局、国家中医药局、中央军委后勤保障部六部门联合发布了我国《第二批罕见病目录》，收录了86种罕见病。目前，两批罕见病目录共收录207种罕见病。

2015年12月24日，国家卫生健康委员会组建了首届罕见病诊疗与保障专家委员会（以下简称"委员会"），并于2020年8月27日对委员会成员进行了更新和扩增，组建了第二届罕见病诊疗与保障专家委员会。第二届委员会由来自罕见病诊疗、医疗保障和社会保障、医学遗传、卫生经济学、公共卫生医学伦理等领域的40位专家组成，涉及从罕见病防治前端的医学研究到后端社会保障等各个方面，标志着我国罕见病防治体系不断向纵深拓展。委员会工作围绕罕见病定义和罕见病目录调整，罕见病防治有关技术规范和临床路径，罕见病预防、筛查、诊疗、用药、康复及保障等方面展开，对加强我国罕见病管理、促进罕见病规范化诊治、保障罕见病用药基本需求、维护罕见病患者健康权益等方面具有重要意义。

2017年10月8日，中共中央办公厅、国务院办公厅印发了《关于深化审评审批制度改革鼓励药品医疗器械创新的意见》，提出支持罕见病治疗药品、医疗器械研发；科学技术部"十三五"国家重点研发计划"精准医学研究"重点专项启动了"罕见病临床队列研究"

与"中国人群重要罕见病的精准诊疗技术与临床规范研究"等课题。以此为开端，中国启动了首个全国性罕见病注册登记研究。作为全国疑难重症诊治中心，北京协和医院牵头此项罕见病临床队列研究，以中国国家罕见病注册系统（National Rare Diseases Registry System，NRDRS）为平台，联合20家国内顶尖教学医院展开研究。目前，该平台登记研究194个研究队列、注册病例超7万例，建设多组学数据库与多中心临床生物样本库，为罕见病精准分型、诊断、治疗和预防提供决策依据。

2019年2月15日，国家卫生健康委员会办公厅印发《关于建立全国罕见病诊疗协作网的通知》，旨在加强我国罕见病管理，提高罕见病诊疗水平。国家卫生健康委员会在全国范围内遴选了一定数量的医院组建罕见病诊疗协作网，建立畅通完善的协作机制，对罕见病患者进行相对集中诊疗和双向转诊，充分发挥优质医疗资源辐射带动作用，提高我国罕见病综合诊疗能力，逐步实现罕见病早发现、早诊断、能治疗、能管理的目标。

2019年2月，受国家卫生健康委员会医政司委托，由中国罕见病联盟和北京协和医院牵头编写的中国首部罕见病诊疗指南《罕见病诊疗指南（2019年版）》发布。该指南对121种罕见病的"概述""病因和流行病学""临床表现""辅助检查""诊断""鉴别诊断""治疗"等进行了全方位阐述，并参考国内外最新的单病种指南诊疗规范和专家共识为每种罕见病附上诊疗流程图，充分展示了该指南对罕见病诊疗实践的规范性、指导性和实用性，对提升我国罕见病规范化诊疗能力具有重要意义。

近年来，我国出台多项纲领政策加速罕见病用药的审评审批和供应保障。2019年12月1日起实施的《中华人民共和国药品管理法》（以下简称"《药品管理法》"）规定，国家鼓励短缺药品的研制和生产，对临床急需的短缺药品、防治重大传染病和罕见病等疾病的新药予以优先审评审批。2021年3月12日，《中华人民共和国国民经济和社会发展第十四个五年规划和2035年远景目标纲要》（以下简称"《纲要》"）发布，《纲要》提出"加快临床急需和罕见病治疗药品、医疗器械审评审批"。2022年5月20日，国务院办公厅印发《"十四五"国民健康规划》，重申对符合要求的罕见病治疗药品加快审评审批的举措。对于罕见病患者群体的用药需求，国家高度重视，相关部门快速响应，建立了罕见病药品供应保障、促进患者药物可及的通道。

"十四五"时期，我国进入高质量发展阶段，罕见病防治与保障事业也迈向新台阶，各级政府对罕见病工作愈发重视。2022年1月30日，工业和信息化部等九部门联合发布的《"十四五"医药工业发展规划》提出重点发展针对罕见病治疗需求，具有新靶点、新机制的化学新药；从审评审批、专利期延长等方面研究制定罕见病药物开发激励政策，落实税费优惠政策，鼓励企业加快相关品种开发；落实研发费用加计扣除和抗癌药品、罕见病药品增值税简易征收等扶持政策，进一步提升财政金融的支持水平。2022年5月10日，国家发展改革委发布《"十四五"生物经济发展规划》，明确提出推动抗体药物、重组蛋白、多肽、细胞和基因治疗产品等生物药发展，鼓励推进慢性病、肿瘤、神经退行性疾病等重大疾病和罕见病的原创药物研发，以提高临床医疗水平。

财政部专门安排资金，切实支持罕见病研究和防治工作开展，自2021年起，中央专项彩票公益金每年支持实施罕见病诊疗水平能力提升项目，截至2023年共安排1.93亿元。相关资金主要用于支持开展疑难罕见病患者多学科诊疗、罕见遗传病患者遗传检测和遗传咨询、医生罕见病诊疗能力培训等，为罕见病防治事业提供了有力保障。

加强罕见病防治工作，既是推动健康中国建设的重要任务，也是全面建成小康社会的必然要求，更是落实党中央、国务院决策部署，造福人民群众的德政工程、民心工程。我国政府一直坚持把人民生命安全和身体健康放在第一位的原则，以人民健康需求为己任，把人民对美好生活的向往作为努力奋斗的目标，坚守对生命的敬畏，履行对健康的承诺，坚定信心，主动作为，不断提升我国的罕见病防治与保障能力，切实维护罕见病患者健康权益，为建设健康中国贡献力量！

第二章　切实加强罕见病预防与诊疗

国家卫生健康委员会始终按照"预防为主、分类施策、稳步推进"的原则，开展罕见病防治管理相关工作。

一、预防为主，降低罕见病发生率

习近平总书记在2016年全国卫生与健康大会上强调，要保障妇幼健康，合理配置服务资源，加强产科、托幼等健康服务供给，倡导优生优育，解决好出生缺陷、营养性疾病、危急重症等威胁妇女和婴幼儿健康的突出公共卫生问题，实施好农村妇女"两癌"筛查，筑牢妇幼健康保障网。

2018年国家卫生健康委员会印发《全国出生缺陷综合防治方案》，作为出生缺陷综合防治的指导性文件，其明确提出通过加强服务网络、人才、经费、科研和信息支撑，做好一级、二级、三级预防，降低出生缺陷发生风险，减少严重出生缺陷和先天残疾发生，规范防治服务。各地陆续印发实施方案，推动任务落实。

2020年，《中华人民共和国基本医疗卫生与健康促进法》（以下简称"《基本医疗卫生与健康促进法》"）正式实施，其第二十四条提出"国家发展妇幼保健事业，建立健全妇幼健康服务体系，为妇女、儿童提供保健及常见病防治服务，保障妇女、儿童健康。国家采取措施，为公民提供婚前保健、孕产期保健等服务，促进生殖健康，预防出生缺陷"。2021年，国务院发布的《中共中央国务院关于优化生育政策促进人口长期均衡发展的决定》，将保障孕产妇和儿童健康、综合防治出生缺陷等作为提高优生优育服务水平的重要内容安排部署；2021年，国务院发布《中国妇女发展纲要（2021—2030年）》，将防治出生缺陷作为重要内容，推进婚前医学检查、孕前优生健康检查、增补叶酸等婚前孕前保健服务更加公平可及，构建完善覆盖婚前、孕前、孕期、新生儿和儿童各阶段的出生缺陷防治体系，预防和控制出生缺陷。为落实《中共中央国务院关于优化生育政策促进人口长期均衡发展的决定》和《中国妇女发展纲要（2021—2030年）》《中国儿童发展纲要（2021—2030年）》要求，进一步完善出生缺陷防治网络，提升出生缺陷防治能力，改善优生优育服务水平，国家卫生健康委办公厅发布《出生缺陷防治能力提升计划（2023—2027年）》，建立覆盖城乡居民，涵盖婚前、孕前、孕期、新生儿和儿童各阶段，更加完善的出生缺陷防治网络，显著提升出生缺陷综合防治能力。到2027年，将实现全国出生缺陷导致的婴儿死亡率、5岁以下儿童死亡率分别降至1.0‰、1.1‰以下。

（一）大力推进一级预防

一方面，有关部门广泛开展社会宣传和健康教育，大力普及优生知识和罕见病相关知识，营造关注罕见病、关爱罕见病患者的社会氛围。在推进婚前保障和孕前优生检查时，将罕见病列入重点，通过病史询问、健康教育等服务，加强针对性咨询指导。实施免费孕前优生健康检查项目，覆盖全国所有县（市、区），为农村计划妊娠夫妇提供19项孕前优生服务，每年有600多万个家庭受益。指导各地遵照《人类辅助生殖技术管理办法》及相关技术规范要求，为有优生需求的罕见病高风险家庭提供胚胎植入前遗传学诊断技术服务，阻断遗传病代际传递。

另一方面，为强化科技支撑，国务院发布《国家中长期科学和技术发展规划纲要（2006—2020年）》，把"出生缺陷防治"列为人口与健康重点领域的优先主题。《"十三五"国家科技创新规划》《"十三五"卫生与健康规划》将"生殖健康及出生缺陷防控研究"纳入国家重点研发计划项目。《"十四五"国民健康规划》指出"实施出生缺陷综合防治能力提升计划，构建覆盖城乡居民，涵盖婚前、孕前、孕期、新生儿和儿童各阶段的出生缺陷防治体系"。2016年以来，国家卫生健康委员会启动出生缺陷防控研究项目52个，不断推动出生缺陷防控科学研究和成果应用转化。

（二）不断强化二级预防

结合孕期保健，广泛开展产前筛查与产前诊断，提高孕期罕见病的发现率和干预率，指导各地根据《产前诊断技术管理办法》及相关技术规范要求，为有罕见病家族史的孕妇提供遗传咨询和产前诊断服务，为有罕见病生育史的计划怀孕夫妇提供遗传咨询等服务，指导夫妇知情选择，采取干预措施。

2019年4月，国家卫生健康委员会第一届全国产前诊断专家组成立，专家组由临床、医学影像、实验室诊断等相关领域的49名专家组成，秘书处设在北京协和医院，为加强产前诊断提供了技术支撑。2020年1月，国家卫生健康委员会印发《开展产前筛查技术医疗机构基本标准》和《开展产前诊断技术医疗机构基本标准》，从主要职责、设置要求、人员能力、房屋与场地、设备配置、规章制度、质量控制等方面对开展产前筛查技术和产前诊断技术的医疗机构提出明确要求，指导各地规范机构设置、完善服务网络。对于常见遗传病，针对携带者筛查的研究陆续在各医疗机构遗传中心开展。

（三）逐步落实三级预防

2009年，卫生部印发《新生儿疾病筛查管理办法》（卫生部令第64号）和《全国新生儿疾病筛查工作规划》，对我国新生儿疾病筛查工作作出总体设计，并对工作目标、组织管理、服务网络、人才队伍、质量管理、科学研究、经费投入等相关方面进行了明确规定。各省（区、市）卫生行政部门根据实际情况，逐步建立起布局合理、系统完善的新生儿疾病筛查网络和信息网络。

财政部门积极支持实施包括贫困地区新生儿疾病筛查在内的基本公共卫生服务项目。自2012年起，卫生计生部门将苯丙酮尿症纳入贫困地区新生儿疾病筛查范围，指导部分省份结合实际将先天性肾上腺皮质增生症等罕见病纳入筛查范围，促进早诊早治。项目的实施，对提高贫困地区新生儿疾病筛查率起到了积极作用，也推动了全国新生儿疾病筛查工作，截至2017年底，全国共有200余家新生儿疾病筛查中心，覆盖全国31个省（区、市），实现了新生儿疾病筛查中心建设的省级全覆盖，健全了省、地市、县三级新生儿疾病筛查网络。

至2022年，全国婚前保健机构、孕前优生健康检查机构已有4000多家，产前筛查机构已达4800多家，产前诊断机构已达498家。

全国有97%的行政区县开展了新生儿疾病筛查工作，有26个省份的全部行政区县都开展了新生儿疾病筛查工作。2018年全国两病（苯丙酮尿症和先天性甲状腺功能减退症）筛查率为98.5%，相比2016年筛查率的97.5%提高了1个百分点。

二、分类施策，解决不同类别罕见病问题

（一）对有治疗或干预手段的罕见病加强诊疗管理

1．初步构建覆盖全国的罕见病防治网络

2019年，国家卫生健康委员会在全国遴选罕见病诊疗经验较多、技术较强的省级及地市级三级医院建立了全国罕见病诊疗协作网（以下简称"协作网"）。协作网包括1家国家级牵头医院、32家省级牵头医院和291家成员医院，基本实现了全国地级市全覆盖。协作网明确了结合分级诊疗制度要求，着力建立协作机制，根据牵头医院和成员医院职责分工，建立完善协作网医院之间双向转诊、专家巡诊、远程会诊的相关标准和管理制度，做到协同高效，实现罕见病患者的筛查、诊断、治疗、康复、随访等就医全过程连续诊疗服务，很大程度上方便了罕见病患者的就医取药。另外，协作网也在提升诊疗水平、保障药品供应、加强科学研究等方面开展相关工作。

为加强罕见病诊疗、提升各医院对罕见病的重视程度，我国多个省市在地方医学会下成立了罕见病相关的专家委员会、学会或学组。中国医院协会罕见病专业委员会、中华医学会罕见病分会等全国性罕见病专业学会和专家委员会相继成立，持续推进罕见病诊疗培训与研究工作。

2．逐步摸清我国罕见病患者数量及分布情况

2019年11月，国家卫生健康委员会委托北京协和医院开发的"中国罕见病诊疗服务信息系统"正式投入使用，全国500多家医院使用该系统进行罕见病病例登记。系统采集了罕见病患者的基本情况、诊疗信息、家族史、诊疗费用和就诊资料等信息。截至2023年8月，该系统共登记约72万例罕见病患者相关信息，确诊的罕见病病例66万例。这些信息对逐步摸清我国罕见病患者数量及分布情况、疾病诊疗、疾病负担和面临困境等情况具有重要意义，也对政府部门制定更加科学合理的政策措施具有重要指导价值，从而帮助罕见病患者获得更好的服务，保障罕见病患者健康权益。

3．稳步提升罕见病诊疗水平

国家卫生健康委罕见病诊疗与保障专家委员会的建立，为罕见病诊疗与保障工作的开展提供了技术支撑。基于《罕见病诊疗指南（2019年版）》，全国罕见病协作网办公室持续推进罕见病规范化诊疗培训，通过建立系统化罕见病培训体系，切实提升了全国罕见病临床诊疗能力。

在国家卫生健康委员会的指导下，由北京协和医院牵头，中国罕见病联盟和全国罕见病诊疗协作网的成员医院组织开展"中央专项彩票公益金支持全国罕见病诊疗水平能力提升项目"（UPWARDS）。项目于2021年至2023年间，由中央专项彩票公益金拨付专项资金1.92亿元，用于罕见病患者及家庭成员遗传检测和咨询、罕见病诊疗能力培训、疑难罕见病多学科诊疗。截至2023年8月底，该项目建立1300余名罕见病临床诊疗专家师资库，累计罕见病经典病例240余例，开展培训340余场，包含全国罕见病诊疗协作网及其他共

3300多家医疗机构医生参与了培训，培训医生超50 000名，并资助了49 028名患者及家庭成员开展了免费基因检测。

4. 建设国家罕见病医学中心，发挥医疗服务辐射能力和影响力

2022年12月27日，国家卫生健康委员会办公厅发布《国家罕见病医学中心设置标准》，从基本要求、医疗服务能力、教学能力、科研能力、承担公共卫生任务和社会公益性任务情况、落实医疗改革相关任务及医院管理情况等方面明确了国家罕见病医学中心的建设标准。依据要求，国家罕见病医学中心应依托罕见病诊治水平突出的三级甲等综合医院，且为省级及以上罕见病医疗质量控制中心依托单位，具备常态化开展罕见病多学科诊疗（multidisciplinary treatment，MDT）工作的能力，具有近3年参与罕见病新药临床试验或开展国际多中心临床研究的资质等。罕见病医学中心的建设有助于提高我国罕见病相关医疗、教学、科研、预防与管理工作，进一步推动优质医疗资源扩容和区域均衡布局，引领医学科学发展和整体医疗服务能力提升，对于我国罕见病防治体系的建设具有重要意义。

5. 提升罕见病诊疗规范化、均质化

2020年11月，受国家卫生健康委员会医政司委托，北京协和医院牵头筹建国家罕见病质控中心，并在2021年第十四个国际罕见病日来临之际正式建成。中心协同各省多家医院的多学科专家团队开展罕见病规范化诊治质控工作，从罕见病组织管理、规范诊疗、质量控制、持续改进四个层面建立相应的组织体系及工作机制，定期发布质控指标和考核结果，为提升我国罕见病诊疗水平与医疗服务质量提供了学术保障和技术支持。

6. 发挥中医药优势提高罕见病诊疗水平

中医药在我国罕见病综合治疗中发挥了独特优势，一方面，相关部门和专家围绕中医治疗具有优势的病种，制定了肝豆状核变性、多发性硬化、视网膜色素变性等中医诊疗方案和临床路径并推广应用；另一方面，在肝豆状核变性、POEMS综合征等罕见病诊疗中，相关部门和专家综合运用中医药物及非药物疗法，提高患者生存质量。

（二）对尚无治疗或干预手段的罕见病加强医学研究

近年来，国家卫生健康委员会联合科学技术部，通过公益性行业科研专项、"重大新药创制"科技重大专项和国家重点研发计划"精准医学研究"重点专项等科技支撑项目，资助了多项罕见病发病机制、临床诊疗和药物研发的科学研究，为推动我国罕见病自主创新和成果转化提供了有力支撑。（详见"第三章不断推进罕见病科学研究"）

（三）多部门综合施策，稳步推进罕见病防治工作

罕见病患者的权益保障涉及多部门，国家卫生健康委员会积极联合科学技术部、国家药品监督管理局、国家医疗保障局、民政部等，在罕见病相关科学研究、药品审评审批及医疗保障等方面均出台了多项政策措施，为罕见病防治营造了良好的政策环境。同时，积极凝聚社会力量，与相关学会及协会、慈善组织等单位积极合作，在推动罕见病的社会认知、公众科普、患者互助等方面发挥了有益作用。

第三章　不断推进罕见病科学研究

开展罕见病相关科学研究，对从根本上推动罕见病防治能力提升具有重要意义。《第一批罕见病目录》的出台，为推动罕见病科研创新奠定了基础，科学技术部也将罕见病相关科学研究纳入国家战略科研项目。为了推动罕见病相关科学研究取得实质性进展，我国采取与国家科技战略布局相一致的方式，既通过国家战略科研项目资助罕见病相关重要科技攻关项目，也通过国家自然科学基金项目从多面上支持罕见病相关的自由探索类研究。

一、战略布局，逐步攻克罕见病重大科技难题

（一）科学技术部部署罕见病重点攻关项目

科学技术部积极贯彻落实党中央、国务院精神，加强罕见病防控技术攻关工作。"十二五"期间，科学技术部依托国家科技支撑计划支持开展中国罕见疾病防治研究与示范，建立了罕见疾病临床资源数据库。"十三五"期间，科学技术部通过国家重点研发计划"精准医学研究"和"生殖健康及重大出生缺陷"重点专项，支持开展罕见病临床队列、中国人群重要罕见病的精准诊疗技术、常见单基因病及基因组病无创产前筛查、新生儿遗传代谢病筛查诊断、儿童重症遗传病、线粒体遗传病的生物技术及药物治疗等研究，累计支

持经费逾2.4亿元。

其中，科学技术部协同国家卫生健康委员会在国家重点研发计划"精准医学研究"重点专项中对罕见病的研究和诊治进行了专门布局。由北京协和医院承担的"罕见病临床队列研究"项目，中国医学科学院基础医学研究所承担的"中国人群重要罕见病的精准诊疗技术与临床规范研究"项目和中国人民解放军总医院承担的"中国重大疾病与罕见病临床与生命组学数据库"项目形成了罕见病全链条创新联盟。2020年9月，科学技术部批准建立疑难重症及罕见病国家重点实验室，依托北京协和医院，开展罕见病基础研究、应用基础研究及高水平学术交流，聚集和培养优秀人才。

2021年，国家自然科学基金委员会生命与医学板块设立"罕见肿瘤研究"专项项目，直接费用总额度约为3000万元。项目基于我国罕见肿瘤研究现状和临床诊疗需求，结合我国罕见肿瘤在流行病学和病因学等方面的特征，以及我国在常见肿瘤研究和诊疗领域雄厚的研究基础，通过资助相关基础研究与临床和转化应用研究的深度整合研究，建立我国罕见肿瘤临床前研究模型，构建罕见肿瘤分子特征图谱，探寻影响罕见肿瘤发生发展的新的靶分子，从而为我国罕见肿瘤临床精准诊疗提供基础。

（二）新药专项布局罕见病药物研发攻关

按照《国家中长期科学和技术发展规划纲要（2006—2020年）》，国家卫生健康委员会等多部门于2008年启动实施了"重大新药创制"科技重大专项，从临床需求出发，重点针对恶性肿瘤、心脑血管疾病等十类（种）重大疾病进展新药研发，并对血友病、重症肌无力、多发性硬化、特发性肺纤维化、肌萎缩侧索硬化症（amyotrophic lateral sclerosis，ALS）、戈谢病等共立项课题十余项，中央资金投入6823万元，支持相关罕见病药物研发。部分课题取得了重要进展，其中特发性肺纤维化用药吡非尼酮胶囊、血友病用药人凝血酶原复合物注射剂及人凝血因子Ⅷ注射剂（冻干）等获得新药证书，填补了相关领域国产药物空白；2018年石药集团研发的ALS治疗药物丁苯酞被美国食品药品监督管理局（Food and Drug Administration，FDA）认定为孤儿药。

（三）中医药布局罕见病防治攻关

2017年科学技术部、国家中医药管理局印发的《"十三五"中医药科技创新专项规划》，将慢性难治性疾病中医药研究纳入国家科技支撑计划、中医药行业科研专项和国家重点研发计划等科技计划，支持中医药治疗重大疾病和罕见病的活性成分等功能研究，为提升罕见病防控提供了有力的科技支撑。

2019年10月，出台的《中共中央国务院关于促进中医药传承创新发展的意见》提出开展防治重大、难治、罕见疾病和新发突发传染病等临床研究。

2022年3月29日，国务院发布《"十四五"中医药发展规划》，提出"开展中医药防治重大、难治、罕见疾病和新发突发传染病等诊疗规律与临床研究"。推进中医药在罕见病诊疗与研究领域的发展，是我国构建罕见病诊疗与保障"中国模式"的特色之路。

二、广泛覆盖，逐步开展罕见病相关自由探索研究

自2016年起，国家自然科学基金委员会设立了"罕见病的发病机制和防治基础研究"专项，鼓励广大科研人员关注人体各系统罕见病的发病机制和防治基础研究。截至2020年，国家自然科学基金委员会已资助罕见病相关研究134项，共涉及人体十多个系统。

第四章 持续提升罕见病药品供应保障水平

我国高度重视罕见病患者用药难题，坚持将罕见病药品上市准入与创新工作纳入国家药品供应保障体系，出台了多项激励政策推动罕见病药物研发和注册上市，包括加快罕见病药品研制进程、提高国家财税政策支持力度、确立罕见病药品优先审评审批制度等，在健全药品供应保障体系中逐步推进罕见病药品可及工作。

一、建立罕见病药品研发创新的法制化保障体系

我国已经形成以《中华人民共和国基本医疗卫生与健康促进法》（以下简称"《基本医疗卫生与健康促进法》"）为核心，以《中华人民共和国药品管理法》（以下简称"《药品管理法》"）为主干，以《药品注册管理办法》《用于罕见病防治医疗器械注册审查指导原则》《临床急需境外新药审评审批工作程序》《接受药品境外临床试验数据的技术指导原则》等为主要支撑的罕见病用药研制保障法律法规体系。其中《基本医疗卫生与健康促进法》明确规定，国家支持防治罕见病药品的研制、生产以满足疾病防治需求;《药品管理法》明确规定，国家鼓励罕见病用药研发，对临床急需的新药予以优先审评审批。

国务院各部委及时发布政策，保障罕见病用药研制活动"与时

俱进"。2015年8月，在国务院出台《关于改革药品医疗器械审评审批制度的意见》后，国家药品监督管理部门成立了药品医疗器械审评审批制度改革领导小组及其办公室，至2016年8月陆续印发了《关于药品注册审评审批若干政策的公告》《关于解决药品注册申请积压实行优先审评审批的意见》等改革配套文件近30项，集中解决包括罕见病用药在内的注册审评积压问题，加快新药审批上市，药品审评审批政策的改革成果已写入2019版《中华人民共和国药品管理法》。

2022年5月9日，《中华人民共和国药品管理法实施条例（修订草案征求意见稿）》首次提出"对批准上市的罕见病新药，在药品上市许可持有人承诺保障药品供应情况下，给予最长不超过7年的市场独占期，其间不再批准相同品种上市"。从审评审批、专利期延长等方面制定罕见病药物开发激励政策，将助力我国建立综合性的罕见病药品研发与诊疗保障体系。

二、国家财税政策支持罕见病药品研发和引进

我国在鼓励本土企业自主开展罕见病药品的创新研发实践中，已经形成了以"财政资助、税收优惠"为核心的财税激励政策。

一是2016年12月财政部发布的《关于"支持和鼓励我国孤儿药发展"建议的答复（摘要）》中，总结了我国对罕见病用药研发创新领域提供税收优惠政策，只要企业符合相关条件，即可享受税收优惠。国家也通过科技计划体系、基本运行经费、基本科研业务费和科技成果转化引导基金对罕见病用药的创新提供支持。

二是在2019年2月召开的国务院常务会议中，决定对首批21个

罕见病药品及其原料药实行降税优惠，参照抗癌药，对进口环节可选择按 3% 征收增值税，国内环节可选择按 3% 简易办法计征增值税；继首批罕见病药品制剂及原料药清单公布实施后，2020 年 9 月和 2022 年 11 月，又发布两批适用增值税政策的罕见病药品清单，截至目前，共计 54 个罕见病药品制剂和 5 个原料药。国家通过多项财税政策的落实，在一定程度上激发了企业对罕见病用药研发投入的热情。

三、审评审批制度改革助力罕见病药品快速上市

一是国家对罕见病用药上市注册予以优先审评审批，获准进入优先审批程序的审评时限为 130 个工作日，其中临床急需境外已上市罕见病用药优先审评审批程序的时限为 70 个工作日。国家进一步落实药品优先审评审批工作机制，与罕见病用药申请人建立沟通交流机制，加强对药品研发的指导，对纳入优先审评审批范围的药品注册申请、审评、检查、审批等各环节优先配置资源，加快审评审批。截至 2023 年 10 月，批准的罕见病药物达到 101 个。

二是附条件上市制度可以让罕见病患者尽早使用已有临床试验数据显示疗效并能预测其临床价值的产品，并要求产品上市后继续开展临床试验确证获益大于风险。

三是鼓励参与国际多中心临床试验，开展境内外同步研发，对符合条件的境外已上市罕见病药品，可以部分甚至全部豁免上市前国内临床试验，直接提交境外取得的临床试验数据申报药品上市注册，大幅缩短罕见病用药在我国上市时间。

四是出台多部技术指导原则。2022 年，国家药品监督管理局药

品审评中心发布多项罕见病药物研发技术指导原则，为罕见病药物的开发提供指导规范，提高研究质量和研发效率。《罕见疾病药物临床研发技术指导原则》《罕见疾病药物临床研究统计学指导原则（试行）》发布，指导原则结合罕见疾病特点，从药物临床研究设计和分析、临床研究实施中的注意事项、证据评价等方面，针对关键统计学问题等方面进行阐述。为推进"以患者为中心"的药物研发，国家药品监督管理局药品审评中心正积极制定相关指导原则，2022年11月，《组织患者参与药物研发的一般考虑指导原则（试行）》正式发布。2023年7月，《以患者为中心的临床试验设计技术指导原则》《以患者为中心的临床试验实施技术指导原则》《以患者为中心的临床试验获益－风险评估技术指导原则》已正式发布实施，推动了以患者为中心理念在药物研发的应用。这些指导原则将从多方面明确患者组织参与药物研发的基本原则，提出临床试验设计、实施、获益－风险评估方面的要求和相关因素考量，鼓励申办者直接组织患者参与药物研发工作。

为推动和规范我国罕见疾病的疾病自然史研究，提供可参考的技术规范，在国家药品监督管理局的部署下，药审中心组织制定了《罕见疾病药物开发中疾病自然史研究指导原则》。

四、罕见病药物卫生技术评估助力罕见病药品可及

卫生技术评估（health technology assessment，HTA）通过对卫生技术的安全性、有效性、经济性和社会性等方面进行全面系统评价，已成为国家和地区决策分析和目录准入管理工具。我国医保药品目录和基本药物目录调整等政策越来越关注药物的卫生技术评估

证据。

然而，传统的评估方法并不完全适用于罕见病治疗技术。对于绝大部分罕见病治疗技术，由于其医疗费用高，临床效果不确定性大和长期疗效证据缺乏等因素，按传统的随机盲法［如随机对照试验（randomized controlled trial，RCT）］等临床试验设计和增量成本-效果比（incremental cost-effectiveness ratio，ICER）分析难以判断罕见病诊治技术价值，限制了对潜在治疗技术的患者可及。鉴于罕见病药物目标患者较少、替代治疗方案有限、普遍成本效益低等，针对罕见病药物的卫生技术评估，中国罕见病联盟组织多学科专家围绕卫生技术评估内涵、评估评审流程与方法、借鉴多维度决策分析（multi-criteria decision analysis，MCDA）原则，制定了《罕见病药物卫生技术评估专家共识（2019版）》。这项工作，为罕见病药物价值判断的流程、方法和标准提供了技术支撑，为中国罕见病药物卫生技术评估指南的形成奠定了基础。目前，《罕见病药品临床综合评价指南》正在编写中。

五、药品供应保障相关举措逐步推进罕见病用药可及

我国已初步建立起一个规范完整的药品供应保障体系，通过体系中关联法律制度间的协同效应，为促进罕见病药品可及提供系统支持。

一是实施符合我国国情的罕见病药物同情用药制度。同情用药制度可以满足罕见病患者预先使用处于临床研究阶段的试验性药物，包括在国外尚未上市的试验性药物。根据《药品管理法》的规定，对正在开展临床试验的用于治疗严重危及生命且尚无有效治

疗手段的疾病的药物，经医学观察可能获益，并且符合伦理原则的，经审查、知情同意后可以在开展临床试验的机构内用于其他病情相同的患者。2021年6月，用于治疗阵发性睡眠性血红蛋白尿症（paroxysmal nocturnal hemoglobinuria，PNH）的Iptacopan成功引进，并在北京协和医院实施，成为我国同情用药的破冰之旅。

二是给予罕见病药品市场独占期。我国正在积极探索实施数据保护制度，2022年5月，国家药品监督管理局发布《中华人民共和国药品管理法实施条例（修订草案征求意见稿）》（以下简称"征求意见稿"）。征求意见稿第四十条"数据保护"，进一步扩大数据保护范围，拟建立"获批上市部分药品""未披露试验数据和其他数据实施保护"的制度，从而进一步深化了2002年以来我国对药品数据保护制度的立法探索。2022年，《中华人民共和国药品管理法实施条例（修订草案征求意见稿）》首次提及对罕见病新药给予最长不超过7年的市场独占期。

三是对于符合条件的临床急需药品开放临时进口的通道。2018年10月，国家药品监督管理局会同国家卫生健康委员会联合发布《关于临床急需境外新药审评审批相关事宜的公告》（2018年第79号），建立专门通道对临床急需境外已上市新药进行审评审批，共遴选发布了三批临床急需境外新药品种名单，鼓励企业申报。三批遴选发布的81个品种中罕见病治疗药品超过50%。目前，已有23个罕见病药品通过临床急需境外新药专门通道获批上市。

2022年6月29日，国家卫生健康委员会和国家药品监督管理局联合印发《临床急需药品临时进口工作方案》和《氯巴占临时进口工作方案》，这两份文件明确了国内无注册上市、无企业生产或短时期内无法恢复生产的境外已上市临床急需少量药品可采用临时进口的方式引进我国，更充分地满足罕见病等重大疾病的临床用药需求。

2022 年 8 月，在北京协和医院牵头下，第一批用于治疗罕见难治性癫痫的进口氯巴占药物进入中国，并于当年 9 月 22 日开出全国首张处方，从此患者可通过遍布全国的 50 家三级医院购买到氯巴占，标志着临床急需药品临时进口通道正式建立，创新了中国特色罕见病药物可及的机制，为其他罕见病药物可及探索了解决路径，同时激励了相关领域的药物研发。2022 年 10 月 22 日，宜昌人福药业有限责任公司的首款国产氯巴占仿制药上市，罕见病药品国产化进程加速。

四是加强包括罕见病用药在内的药品生产监测和保障。2022 年 7 月，工业和信息化部、国家卫生健康委、医保局和药监局联合印发《关于加强短缺药品和国家组织药品集中采购中选药品生产储备监测工作的通知》，建立完善"短缺药品生产供应监测预警平台"，加强对包括罕见病用药在内的重点药品生产、流通、库存等情况开展动态监测和分析预警，强化生产调度和要素保障，对可能出现短缺的药品，"一企一策"解决企业生产中的困难问题，有效提升罕见病用药保障能力。

五是大力支持罕见病用药产业化。工业和信息化、国家发展改革委等部门落实《"十四五"医药工业发展规划》，强化政策协同，大力支持医药工业企业推动罕见病治疗所需创新产品产业化。通过现有资金渠道，加大项目支持力度，推进产业链上下游企业和科研单位加强协作，支持建设罕见病用药生产技术公共平台，开展关键技术产品攻关，补齐产业链关键短板，有效提高罕见病用药产业化。

第五章 稳步建设罕见病保障体系

我国政府高度重视罕见病社会保障工作，不仅体现在政府主导的基本医疗保险、社会保险、社会福利、社会救助等领域，还体现在政府促进的社会慈善、商业保险等多元社会力量的发展。近年来，社会保障工作进展快速，对罕见病社会保障的改革和探索需要更多勇气与担当。

一、罕见病医疗保障

（一）制度政策设置

2020年2月25日，中共中央、国务院印发了《中共中央国务院关于深化医疗保障制度改革的意见》，要求探索罕见病用药保障机制。2021年1月，国家医疗保障局、财政部联合印发了《关于建立医疗保障待遇清单制度的意见》，进一步明确基本医保内涵边界，厘清基本医保和商业健康保险的保障范围。

2021年10月，国务院办公厅印发《关于健全重特大疾病医疗保险和救助制度的意见》，要求根据经济社会发展水平和各方承受能力，探索建立罕见病用药保障机制，整合医疗保障、社会救助、慈善帮扶等资源，实施综合保障。医疗保障部门坚决贯彻落实党中央、国务院决策部署，认真研究解决罕见病患者的医疗保障问题，迄今已建立了统一的城乡居民医保制度，整合各项医疗保障工作管理职能，发挥基本医疗保险、大病保险、医疗救助三重制度保障合力。

一是稳步提高医保待遇水平。目前城镇职工医保、城乡居民医保政策范围内住院费用报销比例分别达到80%和70%左右。城乡居民大病保险已经全面推开，2019年，大病保险起付线降为上年居民人均可支配收入的一半，政策范围内医疗费用支付比例提高到60%，并对贫困人口实行倾斜支付政策。

二是逐步将符合条件的罕见病药品纳入基本支付医保范围。按照《基本医疗保险用药管理暂行办法》，医保药品目录实行每年动态调整，符合条件的药物将按照企业申报、专家评审、谈判准入等程序纳入医保支付范围。进入《第一批罕见病目录》的121种疾病中，对应的多数对症支持性药品和医疗服务项目已纳入医保支付范围。国家医保药品目录调整时重点考虑罕见病等重大疾病用药，为解决罕见病患者的临床用药实际需求，《2022年国家基本医疗保险、工伤保险和生育保险药品目录调整工作方案》进一步向罕见病患者等特殊人群适当倾斜，罕见病用药申报可不受5年内获批的限制。《国家基本医疗保险、工伤保险和生育保险药品目录（2022年）》包含50余种罕见病用药，覆盖27种罕见病，包括特发性肺动脉高压、C型尼曼匹克病、早发型帕金森病、特发性肺纤维化、亨廷顿病等。2021年，治疗脊髓性肌萎缩症（spinal muscular atrophy，SMA）的诺西那生钠注射液从每针近70万元降到3.3万元左右，下降幅度超过95%。通过医保目录准入谈判已累计纳入26种罕见病用药，平均降价超50%。

三是发挥医疗救助托底功能。对纳入低保对象、特困人员、返贫致贫人口范围的罕见病救助对象，国家统筹加大门诊和住院救助力度，符合规定的医疗费用年度救助限额内救助比例约70%，年度救助限额达到3万～5万元。各地还立足医疗救助基金支撑能力和困难群众需求，适度拓展救助对象范围，及时将发生高额医疗费用的罕见病患者家庭纳入救助范围。农村建档立卡贫困人口等救助对象年度救助限额内政策范围内住院费用的救助比例约为70%。通过基本医保、大病保险、医疗救助三重制度综合保障，农村低收入人口医疗费用实际报销比例达到80%左右。2021年4月，国家医疗保障局等七部委发布《关于巩固拓展医疗保障脱贫攻坚成果有效衔接乡村振兴战略的实施意见》，在全面落实大病保险普惠待遇政策基础上，对特困人员、低保对象和返贫致贫人口实施起付线降低50%、报销比例提高5个百分点、逐步取消封顶线的倾斜保障政策。

（二）降低成本举措

2018年以来，国家医疗保障局等部门坚持"招采合一、量价挂钩"的原则，对通过仿制药质量和疗效一致性评价的多家竞争的药品开展药品集中带量采购，包括安立生坦在内的罕见病用药已纳入药品集中带量采购范围，中选价格从每片100元左右下降到每片20元。目前，药品集中带量采购已实现从试点到全国扩围和常态化运行，逐步将更多品种纳入药品集中带量采购，有效挤出药品价格虚高水分。

（三）地方探索经验

我国各地方政府积极探索罕见病的医疗保障路径，通过健全多层次医疗保障制度缓解了本地区内特殊罕见病患者高额医疗费用负担，走出了自己的特色之路，积累了宝贵经验。这些省份结合当地患者患病情况、财政和医保基金承受能力等实际情况对罕见病医疗和社会保障制度进行了探索，并形成了具有各自特点的罕见病保障模式。总之，快速发展并不断完善的多层次社会保障体系，正在为保障罕见病患者有尊严地生存与有希望地生活编织着密厚的安全网。

二、罕见病社会保障

罕见病的社会保障问题一直是罕见病防治事业的核心问题，罕见病的医疗保障问题更是各界关注的焦点。当前，我国已初步建立了完整覆盖罕见病社会保障的法律体系，主要包括《中华人民共和国宪法》《中华人民共和国教育法》《中华人民共和国劳动法》《中华人民共和国社会保险法》《中华人民共和国基本医疗卫生与健康促进法》《中华人民共和国慈善法》《社会救助暂行办法》等，对我国罕见病社会保障的社会保险、社会救助、社会福利等方面均作出了明确安排。但受限于我国经济社会发展水平，我国对罕见病的社会保障仍处于起步阶段，其制度支撑大多融合在面向广大居民的一般性的制度规范中，尚未拥有相对独立、专门、差异化的罕见病社会保障制度。

（一）加大社会救助力度

针对包括罕见病患者在内的低收入或无收入弱势群体的社会救助工作一直是政府工作的重要内容。我国政府的社会救助能力在不断提高，社会救助水平也在不断提升。各地民政部门及时将符合条件的罕见病患者纳入最低生活保障、特困人员救助供养和临时救助范围。为提高遗传代谢病筛查阳性患儿的救助水平，2016年起，国家卫生健康委员会妇幼健康司积极联合中国出生缺陷干预救助基金会等社会组织启动实施出生缺陷救助项目，优先将《第一批罕见病目录》中的甲基丙二酸血症、苯丙酮尿症等20余种罕见病纳入救助范围。截至2020年7月，已救助罕见病患儿3100多名，拨付救助金2900余万元。项目不断扩大患儿疾病救助范围，现已覆盖包括遗传代谢、神经、心血管、消化、皮肤、泌尿生殖、五官、免疫及血液、内分泌代谢等各系统多种罕见病，提高了医疗保障和救助水平，有效减轻了患儿家庭的经济和精神负担。

（二）扩大社会保险覆盖范围

我国社会保险工作通过立法手段，为包括罕见病患者在内的我国居民提供了不断增长的社会保险待遇。2010年出台的《中华人民共和国社会保险法》，为中国社会保险体系的制度建设与系统运行奠定了法律基础。中国已实现了社会保险制度全覆盖，截至2022年底，全国参加基本医疗保险人数为13.45亿人，职工医保参保3.62亿人，居民医保参保9.83亿人。全国参加基本养老保险人数为10.5亿人。其中，有用人单位的罕见病患者按规定从参加职工基本养老保险制度、满足领取条件时享受职工基本养老保险待遇；其他罕见病患者可依据实际情况按规定参加企业职工基本养老保险或城乡居民基本养老保险，符合条件时，享受相应的养老保险待遇。同时，国家通过建立工伤保险和失业保险制度，为包括罕见病患者在内的工伤职工和失业人员建立了富有中国特色的工伤、失业保障体系。

（三）调动社会力量参与

2016年，我国公布实施了《中华人民共和国慈善法》，为我国社会慈善力量助力罕见病社会保障发展提供了新的保障和动力。我国第一个罕见病公益基金是2009年12月23日启动的中华慈善总会罕见病救助公益基金。据不完全统计，截至2015年，我国罕见病公益基金共有20余个，近年来，这一数量还在不断增加。

2021年12月，中国罕见病联盟和中国红十字基金会共同发起的"罕见病共助基金"正式启动，基金不仅致力于开展罕见病患者救助、罕见病知识科普，还将支持罕见病医师培训、支持与罕见病相关的研究与技术开发等相关公益项目。部分罕见病公益基金已经不仅是民间实施、单项救助，同时被纳入地方政府的多方共付罕见病社会保障机制之中。在此过程中，一些患者组织也逐渐发展，具备了一定的影响力和组织能力，如专注ALS的北京东方丝雨渐冻人罕见病关爱中心，以及培育罕见病社群组织的综合性公益组织北京病痛挑战公益基金会等。截至2019年9月，国内已有80余家罕见病公益组织。

（四）促进商业保险补充保障

罕见病的社会保障需要更多社会力量的参与。近年来，各地相继推出与基本医疗保险相衔接的惠民型商业医疗保险产品，部分产品已经探索将少量罕见病药物纳入保障范围。如山东省大多数"惠民保"产品都纳入了罕见病药物的保障，上海于2021年4月发布的

"沪惠保"将3种罕见病的5种高值用药纳入特定高额药品目录，最高可赔付100万元。据中国银行保险监督管理委员会提供数据，在疾病保险方面，目前已有200多种重大疾病保险产品将一些罕见病纳入保障范围之中。在医疗保险方面，多数商业医疗保险产品将罕见病患者医疗费用纳入保障范围，为大病患者提供就医费用保障。这体现了基本医保范围之外的补充保障作用，不仅有助于政府缓解医保支出压力，降低罕见病患者整体治疗花费，而且在力所能及的范围内，帮助罕见病患者获得公平治疗的机会。

第六章 积极参与罕见病防治国际合作

在提升罕见病防治管理能力方面，我国与世界各国保持着紧密的联系，在学习国外先进管理经验的同时，也对外分享我国的做法与心得，共同推动罕见病防治事业的发展。2014年起，我国代表先后参加联合国第一届和第二届罕见病非政府组织委员会会议，学习他国经验，介绍我国罕见病相关政策，展示我国罕见病防治事业的发展成果。我国多所高校和医疗机构积极与国际组织开展罕见病相关研究合作，取得了一系列重大进展。此外，我国多个社会组织积极联合国际组织举办罕见病相关学术研讨会议、患者关爱等活动，极大地提升了社会各界对罕见病的认知水平。

2022年10月中国罕见病大会上，世界卫生组织驻华代表、国际罕见疾病联盟主席、联合国非政府组织罕见疾病委员会等机构代表对我国以目录形式定义罕见病给予高度认可，对探索中国特色罕见病诊疗与保障之路所做的成绩给予充分肯定。

2023年7月15日，"第一届国际医学基因组高峰论坛"在北京成功召开。本次会议由中国罕见病联盟/北京罕见病诊疗与保障学会联合北京瑞洋博惠公益基金会举办，聚焦国内外全基因组测序（whole genome sequencing，WGS）技术领域的最新进展，呈现国内学术成果，研讨行业标准相关建设，为全球基因组学的发展贡献中国力量。

结　束　语

健康是人类的永恒追求。全力维护罕见病患者的健康权益，是全面保障我国人民健康权的重要一环。加强罕见病防治工作，既是推动健康中国建设的重要任务，也是全面建成小康社会的必然要求，更是落实党中央、国务院决策部署，造福人民群众的德政工程、民心工程。相关部门积极贯彻落实党中央、国务院的精神，相继出台罕见病防治与保障相关政策。经过多年的不懈努力，我国罕见病防治事业在政策法规体系、临床诊疗水平、药品供应机制、社会保障体系、重大科研攻关、国际合作交流等方面均取得了明显进展，越来越多的罕见病患者被发现、被治疗、被关爱。

随着我国罕见病防治事业由高速发展期进入精细完善期，进一步完善细化罕见病防治保障政策的顶层设计与法制进程、创新罕见病药品的保障模式、增加对罕见病诊疗技术与药品研发的支持强度、保障罕见病药品的稳定供应、提高国家相关政策的支持力度等一系列工作将成为中国罕见病防治事业的工作重点。

党和国家在罕见病诊疗与保障的道路上积极探索与实践，各级政府将继续秉持高度的责任感和紧迫感，努力做到全方位、全周期保障人民健康，奋力推动卫生与健康事业全面发展。社会各界将持续协同不断完善罕见病诊疗与保障体系的"中国模式"，实现罕见病患者早发现、早治疗、可治疗、可管理、有药用、能负担的美好愿景。

I. Government Attaches Great Importance to the Prevention and Treatment of Rare Diseases

"Health is an inevitable requirement of the promotion of all-round human development, a basic condition for economic and social development, an important symbol of national prosperity, and a common pursuit of the general public." In the 2016 National Conference on Health, President Xi Jinping's important speech profoundly analyzed the significance of the Healthy China Initiative and served as a framework document to guide health-related works in China under new situations. A new strategic deployment and new tasks and missions have been formulated for advancing the Healthy China Initiative in the new era by the 20th National Congress of the Communist Party of China, with an emphasis on "giving strategic priority to ensuring people's health and improving policies on promoting public health". To implement the important statements of President Xi Jinping on health, efforts must be made to improve the diagnostic and treatment ability of rare diseases and to improve equity and quality of medical and health services. Strengthening the prevention and treatment of rare diseases and other major diseases is essential for the well-being of hundreds of millions of people.

Rare diseases are a collective term for uncommon diseases with low incidence, which are generally chronic and often life-threatening. There are more than 7,000 rare diseases identified worldwide, and the number of new rare diseases discovered every year is increasing by 50 to 280. According to estimates, there are approximately 263 to 446 million people globally affected by rare diseases. Among them, approximately 20 million rare disease patients are from China. Less than 10% of those diseases worldwide have approved corresponding treatment options or medications, and most require life-long medication.

In view of the current national reality and the management level of rare diseases, China has not yet defined rare diseases legally, but managed them in the form of list. In May 2018, the National Health Commission (NHC), the Ministry of Science and Technology, the Ministry of Industry and Information Technology, the National Medical Products Administration, and the National Administration of Traditional Chinese Medicine jointly published the *First List of Rare Diseases* in China, covering 121 rare diseases. It was the first time that rare diseases have been "defined" in the form of a list, which is of milestone significance. The diseases enumerated in the list were selected by renowned experts from various fields, based on the disease incidence of the Chinese population, the level of medical technology, the burden of disease, and the security level, with reference to international experience. In the future, relevant departments will update in batches and dynamically improve the list of rare diseases in China. On September 18, 2023, six departments, namely the National Health Commission, the Ministry of Science and Technology, the Ministry of Industry and Information Technology, the National Medical Products Administration, the National Administration of Traditional Chinese Medicine, and the Logistic Support Department of the Central Military Commission, jointly released the List of the Second Batch of Rare Diseases in China, which included 86 rare diseases. At present, a total of 207 rare diseases are included in the two lists of rare disease.

NHC (formerly the National Health and Family Planning Commission) summoned the first group of experts for the Expert Committee on Rare Disease Treatment and Security (hereinafter referred to as the "Committee") on December 24, 2015, and the second group on August 27, 2020. The second group is composed of 40 experts of rare disease diagnosis and treatment, healthcare security and social security, medical genetics, health economics, medical ethics, and other fields, covering all aspects from medical research at the front end of rare disease prevention and treatment to social security at the back end. This marked the continuous expansion of the rare disease prevention and treatment system in China. The work of the Committee is focused on the definition of rare diseases and the adjustment of the rare disease list, technical specification and clinical pathway of rare disease prevention and treatment, as well as prevention, screening, treatment, medication, recovery and security of rare diseases, which is of great significance to the management of rare diseases in China, the standardized diagnosis and treatment of rare diseases, the guaranteed supply of essential medicines for rare diseases, and the safeguard for patients' health-realated rights.

On October 8, 2017, the General Office of the CPC Central Committee and the General Office of the State Council issued the *Opinions on Deepening the Reform of the Evaluation and Approval Systems and Encouraging Innovation of Drugs and Medical Devices*, which proposed to support the research and development of drugs and medical devices for the treatment of rare diseases; the National Key Research and Development Program "Key Project of Precision Medical Research" of the 13th Five-Year Plan of the Ministry of Science and Technology launched the "Clinical Cohort Study on Rare Diseases" and "Research on Precision Treatment Technologies and Clinical Standards for Important Rare Diseases in Chinese Population" , acting as a start for China to initiate the first nationwide research on rare diseases registration. As a national center for diagnosis and treatment of complex and severe diseases, Peking Union Medical College Hospital (PUMCH) took the lead in this clinical cohort study of rare diseases. With the National Rare Diseases Registry System (NRDRS) as the platform, PUMCH joined hands with 20 top teaching hospitals in China to research on more than 70,000 registered cases of over 194 rare diseases, and built a multi-omics database and a multi-center clinical biospecimen bank to provide a basis for accurate typing, diagnosis, treatment and prevention of rare diseases.

On February 15, 2019, the General Office of NHC issued the *Notice on the Establishment of a National Collaboration Network for the Diagnosis and Treatment of Rare Diseases*, aiming at strengthening the management of rare diseases and improving the diagnosis and treatment of rare diseases in China. A certain number of hospitals have been selected nationwide to form a collaboration network for the diagnosis and treatment of rare diseases, to establish a barrier-free and complete collaboration mechanism, to provide relatively centralized treatment and dual referral for patients with rare diseases, to give full play to the exemplary role of high-quality medical resources, to improve the comprehensive diagnosis and treatment capacity of rare diseases in our country, and to gradually achieve the goal of early detection, early diagnosis, effective treatment and effective management of rare diseases.

In February 2019, the first rare disease treatment guideline of China, *Rare Disease Treatment Guideline* (2019 Edition), commissioned by the Medical Administration of NHC and led by the China Alliance for Rare Diseases and PUMCH, was released. The *Guideline* provides a comprehensive description of the overview, etiology and epidemiology, clinical manifestations, auxiliary examinations, diagnosis and differential diagnosis, and treatment of 121 rare diseases. Referring to the latest guidelines, treatment and diagnosis standards, and professional consensus of each single disease at home and abroad, the *Guideline* also includes a diagnosis and treatment flow chart for each rare disease, fully demonstrating the standardization, guidance, and practicality of the guideline for rare disease treatment and practice. The *Guideline* is of great significance to improving the standardized diagnosis and treatment ability of rare diseases in China.

In recent years, a series of policies have been introduced to expedite the review and approval of drugs for rare diseases and ensure a stable medicine supply. The *Drug Administration Law of the People's Republic of China* (hereinafter referred to as the *Drug Administration Law*), which came into effect on December 1, 2019, stipulates that the State encourages research, development and manufacturing of shortage drug, and implements priority review and approval for drugs for urgent clinical needs and new drugs for the prevention and treatment of serious infectious diseases and rare diseases. On March 12, 2021, the *Outline of the 14th Five-Year Plan (2021-2025) for National Economic and Social Development and Vision 2035 of the People's Republic of China* (hereinafter referred to as the *Outline*) was issued. The *Outline* proposed to accelerate review and approval for medicines and medical devices in urgent need for clinical use and for treating rare diseases. On May 20, 2022, the General Office of the State Council issued the *14th Five-Year Plan for National Health*, reaffirming measures to expedite the review and approval of drugs for rare disease treatment that meet the requirements. The State places a high emphasis on the medication needs of the rare disease patient population, and relevant authorities have responded swiftly by establishing channels to ensure the supply of orphan drugs and promote patients' access to these drugs.

The Ministry of Finance has specially arranged funds to effectively support the research, prevention and treatment of rare diseases. Since 2021, MOF has been allocating central lottery public welfare funds annually for upgrading the diagnosis and treatment of rare diseases, with a total amount of 193 million yuan as of 2023. The funds are mainly used to support the multidisciplinary diagnosis and treatment of patients with complex rare diseases, genetic testing and counseling of patients with rare genetic diseases, and training of doctors in the diagnosis and treatment of rare diseases, thus providing a strong guarantee for the cause of rare disease prevention and treatment.

During the 14th Five-Year Plan period, China has entered a stage of high-quality development, and the prevention, treatment, and development of social security system of rare diseases also advanced to a new level. Governments at all levels have been strengthening emphasis on work related to rare diseases. On January 30, 2022, the *14th Five-Year Plan for Pharmaceutical Industry Development* was jointly issued by the Ministry of Industry and Information Technology and nine other departments. This plan outlined key development priorities, emphasizing the development of novel chemical drugs with new targets and mechanisms to meet the treatment needs of rare diseases. Specific measures such as introducing research incentive policies for the development of orphan drugs, spanning review and approval processes, patent term extension, and the implementation of tax and fee incentives to encourage companies to expedite the development of related varieties were introduced. Additionally, the plan emphasized the implementation of policies such as research and development expense deductions, simplified value-added tax collection for cancer drugs and rare disease drugs, further enhancing financial support from the government. On May 10, 2022, the National Development and Reform Commission released the *14th Five-Year Plan for the Development of the Bioeconomy*, which explicitly outlined the promotion of biopharmaceutical development, including antibody drugs, recombinant proteins, peptides, cell and gene therapy products. This plan encouraged the advancement of original drug research and development for major diseases such as chronic diseases, tumors, neurodegenerative diseases, and rare diseases, with the aim of enhancing clinical medical standards.

President Xi Jinping pointed out that prosperity for all is impossible without health for all. Strengthening the prevention and treatment of rare diseases is not only an important task for implementing the Healthy China Initiative, but also an inevitable requirement for building a moderately prosperous society at all respects, and a benevolent and popular project to implement the decisions of the CPC and the State Council for the benefits of the people. The Chinese government has always adhered to the principle of putting people's safety and health in the first place, taking people's health needs as its responsibility, taking people's aspirations for a better life as the goal to strive for, holding fast to the respect for life, fulfilling the commitment to health, and acting with confidence and initiative to continuously improve the prevention, treatment and social security of rare diseases in China, thus making new contributions to improving the health of the Chinese population and building a well-off society. We will make new and greater contributions to promoting the health of all people and to building a Healthy China!

II. Effective Improvement of the Prevention and Treatment of Rare Diseases

NHC has been upholding the principle of "prevention as priority and categorized policies for steady progress" in carrying out works related to the prevention, treatment and management of rare diseases.

1. "Prevention as priority" for reduced incidence of rare diseases

At the 2016 National Conference on Health, President Xi Jinping noted the importance of protecting the health of women and children and establishing a robust healthcare safety net for women and children. He underscored the need for the rational allocation of service resources, strengthening the supply of obstetrics, childcare and other health services, emphasizing the importance of bearing and rearing better children, and effectively addressing prominent public health issues that threaten the health of women and infants, such as birth defects, nutritional diseases, and critical illnesses. He also emphasized the importance of the implementation of cervical and breast cancer screenings for women in rural areas.

In 2018, the NHC issued the *National Comprehensive Prevention and Control Program for Birth Defects*, which serves as a guiding document for comprehensive birth defect prevention and control, specifying the importance of strengthening service networks, human resources, funding, scientific research, and information support. The program aimed to enhance primary, secondary, and tertiary prevention, reduce the risk of birth defects, minimize the occurrence of severe birth defects and congenital disabilities, and standardize prevention and treatment services. Subsequently, regions across the country issued and implemented their respective action plans to facilitate the realization of these objectives.

In 2020, the *Basic Healthcare and Health Promotion Law of the People's Republic of China* (hereinafter referred to as the *Basic Healthcare and Health Promotion Law*) took effect officially. Article 24 thereof stipulates that "the State develops the cause of maternal and child health maintenance, establishes and improves a maternal and child health service system, and provides women and children with health maintenance and common disease prevention and treatment services, to safeguard the health of women and children and the state adopts measures to provide citizens with pre-marital health maintenance, maternal health maintenance, and other services to promote reproductive health and prevent birth defects." In 2021, the *Decision to Improve Birth Policies to Promote the Long-Term Balanced Development of Population* was issued by the State Council, in which safeguarding the health of pregnant women and children, as well as comprehensive prevention and control of birth defects, were designated as important components to enhance the quality of services related to healthy births. Also in 2021, the State Council released the *Outline for Women's Development in China* (2021-2030), which noted the significance of prevention and treatment of birth defects, the promotion of fairness and accessibility of premarital medical examination, prenatal physical examination, folic acid supplementation and other premarital and prenatal health care services, and advocated building a birth defect prevention and control system covering all stages of pre-marriage, pre-pregnancy, pregnancy, newborns and child care to prevent and control birth defects. To implement the *Decision to Improve Birth Policies to Promote the Long-Term Balanced Development of Population*, the *Outline for Women's Development in China (2021-2030)*, and the *Outline for Children's Development in China (2021-2030)*, and to further improve the network for birth defect prevention and control, as well as to enhance the capacity for birth defect prevention and control, and improve the quality of services related to healthy births, the General Office of the NHC issued the *Plan for Enhancing Birth Defect Prevention and Control Capacity* (2023-2027). This plan aims to establish a more comprehensive birth defect prevention and control network that covers both urban and rural residents and spans various stages from premarital, prenatal, pregnancy, newborn, to childhood, with the expectation of significantly enhancing the comprehensive capability to prevent and control birth defects. By

2027, the national infant mortality rate and the mortality rate of children under 5 years old caused by birth defects will be reduced to below 1.0‰ and 1.1‰ respectively.

(1) Great efforts have been devoted to primary prevention

For one thing, extensive health education and information campaigns have been launched by relevant government departments to popularize knowledge of healthier births and rare diseases, and to raise social awareness of rare diseases and care for patients living with rare diseases. Rare diseases have been incorporated as a key item in premarital health care and pregestational screening. In addition, the implementation of a free pregestational screening program, covering all counties (cities, districts) nationwide, offers 19 pregestational health services to couples in rural areas planning to have children, benefiting over 6 million families annually. All localities have been instructed to provide technical services of preimplantation genetic diagnosis (PGD) in compliance with the *Measures for the Administration of Assisted Reproductive Technology of Human* and related technical specifications for families at high risks of rare diseases preparing for childbirth to interrupt the intergenerational transmission of genetic diseases.

For another, to strengthen technological support, the State Council issued the *Outline of the National Medium- and Long-Term Science and Technology Development Plan* (2006-2020) listing "Birth Defect Prevention and Control" as a priority topic in the field of population and health research. The *National 13th Five-Year Plan for Science and Technology Innovation* and the *National 13th Five-Year Plan for Sanitation and Health* included "Reproductive Health and Birth Defect Prevention and Control Research" as part of the national key research and development projects. The *National 14th Five-Year Plan for Health* points out that "implement the comprehensive birth defect prevention and control ability enhancement plan, and build a birth defect prevention and control system covering urban and rural residents, covering all the stages of pre-marital, pre-pregnancy, pregnancy, neonatal and childhood". Since 2016, the NHC has initiated 52 research projects on birth defect prevention and control, continuously advancing scientific research and the application of results in the field of birth defect prevention and control.

(2) Continuous progresses have been recorded in strengthening secondary prevention

In addition to peri-conception care, prenatal screening and prenatal diagnosis have been widely carried out to improve the detection rate and intervention rate of rare diseases during pregnancy. All localities have been instructed to provide genetic counseling and prenatal diagnosis services for pregnant women with family history of rare diseases, and genetic counseling and other services for couples with history of rare diseases planning to become pregnant, and guide couples to make informed choices and take intervention measures in accordance with the

Measures for the Administration of Prenatal Diagnosis Technology and relevant technical specifications.

In April 2019, the first national expert group for prenatal diagnosis of the NHC was established, consisting of 49 experts from clinical medicine, medical imaging, laboratory diagnostics and other related fields, with the secretariat located at the PUMCH, which provides technical support for strengthening prenatal diagnosis. In January 2020, the NHC issued the *Basic Standards for Medical Institutions Performing Prenatal Screening Technology* and the *Basic Standards for Medical Institutions Performing Prenatal Diagnostic Technology*, which outlined specific requirements for medical institutions performing prenatal screening and prenatal diagnostic technologies, covering key responsibilities, facility requirements, personnel qualifications, premises and locations, equipment, regulations, quality control, and more. They serve as guidelines for standardizing the establishment of institutions and improving service networks across different regions. Furthermore, research on carrier screening for rare genetic diseases that commonly occur has been progressively carried out in genetic centers within various medical institutions.

(3) Steady advancement has been achieved in improving tertiary prevention

In 2009, the former Ministry of Health issued the *Administrative Measures for the Screening of Diseases of New-born Babies* (Order

No. 64 of the Ministry of Health) and *Work Plan for National Neonatal Disease Screening*. These documents put forward the overall design of the neonatal disease screening in China, and clearly defined the work objectives, management of organizations, service network, talent team, quality management, scientific research, fund investment and other relevant aspects. Administrative departments of health and family planning of all provinces, autonomous regions and municipalities directly under the central government have gradually established neonatal disease screening network and information network with reasonable layout and complete system.

The financial organs have actively supported the basic public health service programs, including newborn disease screening in impoverished areas. Since 2012, the health administrative department has included phenylketonuria in neonatal screening in impoverished areas and has provided guidance to some provinces to incorporate other rare diseases such as congenital adrenocortical hyperplasia into the scope of neonatal screening to ensure diagnosis and treatment. This project has played a positive role in improving the screening rate for neonatal diseases in impoverished areas and has also propelled nationwide efforts in neonatal screening. By the end of 2017, there were over 200 neonatal disease screening centers nationwide, covering 31 provinces (districts, municipalities), achieving provincial-level full coverage in the construction of neonatal disease screening centers and establishing a well-rounded neonatal disease screening network at the provincial, municipal, and county levels.

As of 2022, there are over 4,000 premarital healthcare institutions and pregestational screening institutions nationwide, with more than 4,800 prenatal screening institutions and 498 prenatal diagnostic institutions. Neonatal disease screening was carried out in 97% of districts and counties nationwide; and 26 provinces achieved full coverage of neonatal disease screening in all counties within their jurisdictions. The national screening rate for phenylketonuria and congenital hypothyroidism was 98.5% in 2018, increasing by 1% from 97.5% in 2016.

2. Targeted measures for rare diseases of different categories

(1) Strengthened diagnosis and treatment for rare diseases with proven treatment or intervention measures

a. Initial progresses in establishing a nationwide prevention and treatment network.

In 2019, the NHC has selected hospitals with abundant experience and leading technological capacity in rare disease diagnosis and treatment to form a national collaboration network for rare disease diagnosis and treatment. The three-level network is composed of one leading national hospital, 32 provincial hospitals and 291 member hospitals, basically achieving full prefecture-level coverage. The collaboration network has established a collaboration mechanism in accordance with the tiered diagnosis and treatment system; relevant standards and management systems for dual referral, specialist rounds and remote consultation among the hospitals within the collaboration network have been established and improved according to the division of responsibilities between the lead hospital and member hospitals, so as to achieve synergy and efficiency, to provide diagnostic and treatment services for patients diagnosed with rare diseases in the whole process of screening, diagnosis, treatment, recovery and follow-up, and to improve accessibility of medicines and medical services for patients with rare diseases. In addition, the collaboration network is also dedicated to improving the diagnosis and treatment capacity, ensuring the supply of drugs, and strengthening scientific research.

In order to strengthen diagnosis and treatment of rare diseases and raise awareness of rare diseases in various hospitals, expert committees, societies, or groups related to rare diseases have been established under local medical associations in several provinces and cities in China. National-level rare disease professional societies and expert committees, such as, the Rare Disease Professional Committee of the Chinese Hospital Association, and the Rare Disease Branch of the Chinese Medical Association, have also been established. These organizations work continuously to promote training and research in the field of rare disease diagnosis and treatment.

b. Understanding of demographic characteristics and distribution of rare diseases in China

In November 2019, the China Information System of Rare Disease Diagnosis and Treatment Services, developed by PUMCH and authorized by NHC, was officially put into use. Up to date, nearly 500 hospitals nationwide now register rare disease cases on this system. The system collects information such as personal profile of patients, diagnostic and treatment information, family history, treatment expense and consultation information. As of August 2023, the system had collected about 720,000 entries of rare disease patients, with 660,000 rare disease cases having been diagnosed. The information is of great significance for understanding the number and distribution of rare disease patients, diagnosis and treatment, disease burdens and problems in China and will also help government departments formulate science-based and reasonable policies and measures to help patients access quality services, and protect their health-related rights.

c．Steady progresses in rare disease diagnosis and treatment.

To improve the standardized diagnosis and treatment of rare diseases in China, ensure medical quality and safety, and safeguard the health rights and interests of patients with rare diseases, the National Health Commission and other four departments issued the the List of the First Batch of Rare Diseases in China and worked with the Expert Committee on Diagnosis, Treatment and Support of Rare Diseases of the National Health Commission (Peking Union Medical College Hospital of Chinese Academy of Medical Sciences) to formulate the Guidelines for the Diagnosis and Treatment of Rare Diseases (2019 edition).

Under the guidance of the NHC and led by PUMCH, in collaboration with the China Alliance for Rare Diseases and member hospitals of the national collaboration network for rare disease diagnosis and treatment, the *Peking Union Medical College Hospital Public Welfare Project for Rare Disease Service Improvement* (UPWARDS) has been initiated. Between 2021 and 2023, 193 million yuan from the Central Lottery Public Welfare Fund has been allocated for genetic testing and counseling of patients with rare diseases and their family members, training of doctors in the diagnosis and treatment of rare diseases, and multidisciplinary diagnosis and treatment of complex rare diseases. As of the end of August 2023, the project has established a talent pool of over 1,300 clinical experts in rare diseases, has accumulated more than 240 classic rare disease cases, and has conducted over 340 training sessions involving doctors from over 3,300 medical institutions, with more than 50,000 doctors benefiting from the training. Additionally, the project has provided free genetic testing for 49,028 patients and their family members.

d. Progresses in establishing a National Rare Disease Medical Center, leveraging the radiating capacity and influence of medical services.

On December 27, 2022, the General Office of the NHC issued the *Establishment Standards for National Rare Disease Medical Centers*, which clarified the construction standards for national rare disease medical centers in terms of the basic requirements, medical service capabilities, teaching capabilities, scientific research capabilities, the fulfillment of public health tasks and social welfare tasks, implementation of tasks related to healthcare reform and hospital management. According to these requirements, national rare disease medical centers should rely on Class A tertiary comprehensive hospitals with outstanding rare disease diagnosis and treatment capabilities, be the relying unit of the medical quality control center for rare diseases at the provincial level and above, have the ability to carry out Multidisciplinary Diagnosis and Treatment (MDT) of rare diseases on a regular basis, and have the qualification to participate in the clinical trial of new drugs for rare diseases or carry out the international multi-center clinical research in the recent three years. The establishment of these medical centers will help improve the medical treatment, teaching, scientific research, prevention and management of rare diseases in China, further promote the expansion of high-quality medical resources and the balanced layout of the region, and lead the development of medical science and the enhancement of the overall medical service capacity, which is of great significance for the construction of China's rare disease prevention and treatment system.

e. Enhancement of standardizing and homogenizing rare disease diagnosis and treatment.

In November 2020, commissioned by the Department of Medical Administration of the National Health Commission, Peking

Union Medical College Hospital took the lead in preparing for the establishment of the National Medical Service Quality Control Center for Rare Diseases, which was completed in 2021 on 14th Rare Disease Day. The center collaborates with multidisciplinary expert teams from various provinces and hospitals to carry out standardized quality control for rare disease diagnosis and treatment. At four different levels, namely rare disease organization and management, standardized diagnosis and treatment, quality control, and continuous improvement, the center has established corresponding organizational structures and working mechanisms and has regularly published quality control indicators and assessment results, providing academic support and technical assistance to enhance China's rare disease diagnosis and treatment standards and healthcare service quality.

f. Traditional Chinese medicine (TCM) for improved diagnosis and treatment of rare diseases.

TCM has played a unique role in the comprehensive treatment of rare diseases in China. For one thing, experts and departments have formulated TCM diagnosis and treatment programs and clinical pathways for Wilson's disease, multiple sclerosis and retinitis pigmentosa and popularized their application; for another, in the diagnosis and treatment of rare diseases such as hepatomegaly and POEMS syndrome, these experts and departments have integrated the use of traditional Chinese drugs and non-pharmacological therapies to improve the quality of life of the survived patients.

(2) Strengthened medical research on rare diseases for which there is no proven treatment or intervention measures yet

In recent years, NHC, together with departments of science and technology, has funded scientific researches on the pathogenesis of rare diseases, clinical treatment and drug discovery, etc. Funding has been provided for scientific research projects such as Special Projects for Public Welfare Industries, Major Projects for New Drugs R&D, and Key Projects for Precision Medicine Research under the National Key Research and Development Program. The funding greatly boosted independent innovation on rare diseases and achievement transformation in China. (For more details, see "III. Continuous Advancement of Scientific Research on Rare Diseases")

(3) Inter-departmental coordinated mechanism yielded steady outcomes in rare disease prevention and treatment

Given the fact that the protection of rights and interests of patients with rare diseases involves various departments, NHC has actively joined hands with other central departments, such as the Ministry of Science and Technology, the National Medical Products Administration, the National Healthcare Security Administration,, and the Ministry of Civil Affairs, to introduce a number of policies and measures concerning scientific research on rare diseases, review and approval of drugs for rare diseases, and medical insurance for rare diseases, etc. In addition to favorable policies for the prevention and treatment of rare diseases, attempts have also been made to gather social forces and unite related academic associations and charitable organizations, which has played a useful role in raising social awareness of rare diseases, and encouraging patients with rare diseases to support each other.

III. Continuous Advancement of Scientific Research on Rare Diseases

Conducting scientific researches on rare diseases is of great significance to fundamentally improving the prevention and treatment of rare disease. The *List of First Batch of Rare Diseases* has laid a foundation for encouraging scientific researches and innovation in the field of rare diseases. The Ministry of Science and Technology has also included scientific researches on rare diseases in the national strategic scientific research projects. In order to encourage substantial progresses in scientific research on rare diseases, China has adopted an approach consistent with the national strategic layout for science and technology, i.e., funding major science and technology research projects related to rare diseases through the national strategic scientific research projects and supporting free exploration and research on rare diseases through the National Natural Science Foundation of China (NSFC).

1. Overcome major scientific and technological problems of rare diseases step by step through strategic layout

(1) The Ministry of Science and Technology deploys key research projects

The Ministry of Science and Technology has actively implemented the spirit of the CPC Central Committee and the State Council to strengthen researches and development of rare disease prevention and control technologies. During the 12th Five-Year Plan period, the Ministry of Science and Technology supported researches and demonstration projects of rare disease prevention and control in China and established the clinical resource database of rare diseases through the National Science and Technology Support Program. During the 13th Five-Year Plan period, the Ministry of Science and Technology, through the National Key R&D Program, specifically the "Precision Medicine Research" and "Reproductive Health and Major Birth Defects", have provided support for the researches on clinical cohorts for rare diseases, precision diagnosis and treatment technologies for important rare diseases in Chinese people, non-invasive prenatal screening (NIPC) for common monogenetic diseases and genomic diseases, screening and diagnosis of neonatal genetic metabolic diseases, severe genetic diseases in children, and mitochondrial genetic diseases, among other biotechnology and pharmaceutical R&D projects, with total funds of about 240 million yuan.

The Ministry of Science and Technology, in collaboration with NHC, has made special arrangements for the researches and treatment of rare diseases in "Precision Medicine Special Projects" of the National Key R&D Program. The "Clinical Cohort Study of Rare Diseases" undertaken by PUMCH, the "Research on Precision Diagnosis and Clinical Standardization of Important Rare Diseases in Chinese Population" undertaken by the Institute of Basic Medical Sciences of the Chinese Academy of Medical Sciences, and the project of "Clinical and Life Cycle Database of Major Diseases and Rare Diseases in China" undertaken by the General Hospital of the People's Liberation Army have formed a whole chain of innovation alliance for rare diseases. In September 2020, the Ministry of Science and Technology approved the establishment of the State Key Laboratory of Difficult Severe and Rare Diseases, in collaboration with PUMCH, to carry out basic research, applied basic research and high-level academic exchanges on rare diseases, as well as to gather and cultivate talents.

In 2021, the Life and Medicine Sector of the National Natural Science Foundation of China set up a special project named "Rare Tumor Research", with a total direct budget of about 30 million yuan. Based on the current situation of rare tumor research and clinical diagnosis and treatment needs in China, combining the characteristics of rare tumors in epidemiology and etiology, as well as China's research foundation in the field of common tumor research and diagnosis and treatment, the project aims to establish a preclinical research model of China's rare tumors by funding the in-depth integration of relevant basic research with clinical and translational application research, constructing a molecular profiles of rare tumors, and exploring new target molecules affecting the development of rare tumors, thereby laying the foundation of clinical precision diagnosis and treatment of China's rare tumors.

(2) New drug special projects for rare disease research and development

In accordance with the *Outline of the National Medium- and Long-Term Science and Technology Development Plan* (2006-2020), multiple departments such as the NHC initiated Major Science and Technology Special Projects of Major New Drug R&D in 2008, focusing on clinical needs and support researches on and development of new drugs for 10 types of major diseases, such as malignant tumor, cardiovascular diseases, as well as other diseases such as hemophilia, myasthenia gravis, multiple sclerosis, idiopathic pulmonary fibrosis, amyotrophic lateral sclerosis (ALS), Gaucher's disease, etc. The central government has invested 68.23 million yuan to support R&D of rare diseases. Some of the projects have already yielded preliminary outcomes, among which pirfenidone capsules for idiopathic pulmonary fibrosis, human prothrombin complex injection and human coagulation factor injection (lyophilized) for hemophilia have obtained new drug certificates, filling the gaps of domestic drugs in these fields. In 2018, butylphthalide for

ALS developed by CSPC Pharmaceutical Group Co., Ltd. was defined as an orphan drug by the U.S. Food and Drug Administration (FDA).

(3) TCM supports research on the prevention and treatment of rare diseases

In 2017, the Ministry of Science and Technology and the National Administration of TCM issued the *13th Five-Year Plan for TCM Science and Technology Innovation*, which proposed to support TCM researches on chronic and intractable diseases through the National Science and Technology Support Program, the Special Research Projects for TCM Industry, the National Key R&D Program and functional research on active constituents in the treatment of major diseases and rare diseases. These researches provide a strong scientific and technological support for the prevention and control of rare diseases.

In October 2019, a *Guideline on Promoting the Inheritance, Innovation and Development of Traditional Chinese Medicine* issued by the General Office of the CPC Central Committee and the General Office of the State Council proposed to carry out clinical research on the prevention and treatment of major, intractable, and rare diseases, as well as new and outbreaks of infectious diseases.

On March 29, 2022, the State Council issued the *14th Five-Year Plan for the Development of Traditional Chinese Medicine*, which states that "carrying out clinical research on the diagnosis and treatment patterns of traditional Chinese medicine for the prevention and treatment of major, intractable and rare diseases, as well as new and outbreaks of infectious diseases." This plan also aims to promote the development of traditional Chinese medicine in diagnosis, treatment and research of rare diseases, contributing to the establishment of a distinctive "Chinese model" for rare disease diagnosis, treatment, and support.

2. Extensive explorations and researches on rare diseases

Since 2016, NSFC has established the special project on "Basic Research on the Pathogenesis and Prevention of Rare Diseases" to encourage researchers to focus on basic researches on the pathogenesis and prevention of rare diseases in various human body systems. As of 2020, NSFC has funded 134 studies related to rare diseases, involving more than 10 human body systems.

IV. Continuous Improvement of Supply of Orphan Drugs

China attaches great importance to the accessibility of medication for patients with rare diseases, and insists on incorporating market access and innovation of orphan drugs into the national drug supply security system. A number of incentive policies have been introduced to promote R&D and registration of orphan drugs, including acceleration of drug R&D, increased national financial and tax policy support, and priority review and approval system for orphan drugs. These measures will gradually improve the accessibility of orphan drugs while improving the drug supply system.

1. Establishment of law-based guarantee framework for R&D of orphan drugs

China has established a legal framework to safeguard the R&D of drugs for rare diseases, including laws and regulations such as the *Law of the People's Republic of China on the Promotion of Basic Medical and Health Care* (hereinafter referred to as the Basic Medical and Health Care Promotion Law), *Pharmaceutical Administration Law of the People's Republic of China* (hereinafter referred to as the Pharmaceutical

Administration Law), *Measures for the Administration of Drug Registration, Guiding Principles for Registration and Review of Medical Devices for Prevention and Treatment of Rare Diseases, Procedures for Review and Approval of Clinically Urgent New Overseas Drugs,* and *Technical Guidelines for Receiving Overseas Clinical Trial Data of Drugs. The Basic Medical and Health Care Promotion Law* clearly stipulates that the State shall support the research, development, and production of drugs for prevention and of rare diseases to meet the needs of disease prevention and control; the Pharmaceutical Administration Law clearly stipulates that the State shall encourage the development of new drugs for rare diseases and give priority to the review and approval of drugs in urgent clinical needs.

Ministries of the State Council issued policies in a timely manner to ensure that R&D of drugs could "keep pace with the times". In August 2015, after the State Council issued the *Opinions on the Reform of the Review and Approval System of Drugs and Medical Devices*, the National Medical Products Administration established a leading group and office for the reform of the review and approval system of drugs and medical devices, and by August 2016, some 30 supporting documents such as the *Announcement of Certain Policies on the Review and Approval of Drug Registration* and the *Opinions on Giving Priority to Review and Approval to Solve the Backlog of Drug Registration Applications* were issued successively to deal with the backlog of registration review. Reform outcomes, such as the policy to accelerate the approval of new drugs have been incorporated into the 2019 Pharmaceutical Administration Law.

On May 9, 2022, for the first time, the *Implementation Regulations of the Drug Administration Law (Draft Revisions)* introduced the concept of "granting a market exclusivity period of up to 7 years for approved new drugs for rare diseases, provided that the drug's marketing authorization holder commits to ensuring drug supply. During this period, no approvals for the same drug category shall be granted" . This initiative, which encompasses incentives for R&D of orphan drugs in aspects such as review and approval, and patent term extension, will contribute to the establishment of a comprehensive guarantee framework for R&D of drugs and therapies for rare diseases in China.

2. National financial and tax policy for R&D and introduction of orphan drugs

China has developed a financial and tax incentive policy, i.e., "financial support and preferential tax" , to encourage local enterprises to carry out R&D of orphan drugs.

First, the *Reply to the Proposal of "Supporting and Encouraging the Development of Orphan Drugs in China" (Abstract)*, released by the Ministry of Finance in December 2016, summarized that China had been providing tax incentives for the R&D and innovation of orphan drugs, and enterprises can enjoy tax incentives as long as they meet the relevant requirements. China also provides support for innovation in orphan drugs by means of science and technology planning, basic operating funds, basic scientific research operating expenses and the National Fund for Technology Transfer and Commercialization.

Second, in the executive meeting of the State Council held in February 2019, it was decided that the first list of 21 orphan drugs and their active pharmaceutical ingredients (APIs) would be subject to a tax reduction, with reference to anti-cancer drugs for which the import link may choose to levy value-added tax (VAT) at 3% and the domestic link may choose to levy VAT at 3% on a simplified basis; following the announcement and implementation of the first list of orphan drug preparations and APIs, two additional lists of orphan drugs were released in September 2020 and November 2022. As of the present, there are a total of 54 orphan drug preparations and 5 APIs included in these lists. The State has, to a certain extent, stimulated enterprises to invest more in the R&D of orphan drugs through the implementation of a number of fiscal policies.

3. Reform of the review and approval system to accelerate marketing of orphan drugs

First, China has prioritized registration review and approval of orphan drugs. The maximum duration for drugs in priority approval process is 130 working days, while the time limit for review of overseas orphan drugs catering to urgent clinical needs is 70 working days. China further implements the priority review and approval mechanism for drugs, establishes a communication mechanism with applicants for orphan drugs, strengthens guidance on drug R&D, and prioritizes the allocation of resources at every stage of drug registration, including review, inspection, and approval, so as to speed up the process. As of 2023, 101 drugs for rare diseases have been approved.

Second, the conditional marketing policy allows patients with rare diseases to use medicine as early as possible whose efficacy has been proved by clinical data and clinical value can be predicted. Post-marketing clinical trials are required to confirm that the medicine's benefits outweigh its risks.

Third, we will encourage participation in international multi-center clinical trials, and carry out simultaneous research and development within and outside the country. We can partially or even completely exempt eligible overseas marketed rare disease drugs from pre-marketing clinical trials in China, and directly submit clinical trial data obtained overseas to declare the drugs for marketing and registration, so as to significantly shorten the time for rare disease drugs to be marketed in China.

Fourth, multiple technical guidance principles have been released. In 2022, the Drug Evaluation Center of National Medical Products Administration issued several technical guidance principles for R&D of orphan drugs, which provide standardized guidance for orphan drug development, aiming to enhance research quality and efficiency. The *Technical Guidance Principles for Clinical Development of Orphan*

Drugs and the *Statistical Guidance Principles for Clinical Research of Orphan Drugs (Trial)*, tailored to the characteristics of rare diseases, have been published to address key statistical issues and provide insights into various aspects, including drug clinical research design and analysis, precautions during clinical research implementation, and evidence evaluation. To advance "patient-centered" drug development, the Drug Evaluation Center of the National Medical Products Administration is actively developing relevant guidance principles. In November 2022, the *General Considerations for Organizing Patient Participation in Drug Development (Trial)* was officially released. In July, 2023, the *Patient-Centered Clinical Trial Design Technical Guidance Principles*, the *Patient-Centered Clinical Trial Implementation Technical Guidance Principles*, and the *Benefit-Risk Assessment Technical Guidance Principles for Patient-Centered Clinical Trials* XX have been put in place, which promotes the patient-centered approach in drug research and development. These guidance principles aim to define the fundamental principles of patient organization involvement in drug development, outline requirements and considerations in clinical trial design, implementation, benefit-risk assessment, and encourage applicants to directly involve patients in drug development.

To promote and standardize the natural history study of rare diseases in China, and to provide technical specifications that can be referred to, the National Medical Products Administration formulated and issued the Guiding Principles for the Natural History Study of

Disease in Developing Rare Disease Drugs.

4. Health technology assessment of orphan drugs help improve accessibility of orphan drugs

Health Technology Assessment (HTA) refers to the comprehensive and systematic evaluation of the safety, effectiveness, and socio-economic effects of health technologies. HTA has become a management tool for national and regional decision analysis and catalog access. The Chinese government pays more attention to HTA evidence when adjusting policies such as the list of reimbursed drugs and the list of essential medicines.

However, traditional assessment approaches sometimes are not suitable for assessing rare disease treatments. Most technologies for the treatment of rare diseases are burdened with high medical costs, uncertain clinical outcomes and the lack of long-term evidence of efficacy. Therefore, it is difficult to determine the value of these technologies for the diagnosis and treatment of rare diseases using traditional clinical trial designs such as randomized controlled trials (RCTs) and incremental cost-effectiveness ratio (ICER) analysis. As a result, patients'accessibility to potential treatment technologies is restricted. In view of the small group of target patients, limited alternative treatment options, and low costeffectiveness of orphan drugs, the China Alliance for Rare Diseases has organized multidisciplinary experts to formulate the *Expert Consensus on Health Technology*

Assessment of Orphan Drugs (2019), which focuses on the significance of HTA, assessment process and methodology, and the principles of Multi-Criteria Decision Analysis (MCDA). This work, which provides technical support for the process, methods and standards for judging the value of drugs for rare diseases, lays the foundation for the guidelines for health technology assessment of drugs for rare diseases in China. Currently, the *Guidelines for Comprehensive Clinical Evaluation of Orphan Drugs* are under development.

5. Relevant measures ensuring drug supply for better accessibility of orphan drugs

China has recorded initial success in establishing a standardized and complete system to improve drug supply. Various laws and regulations have generated a synergy and provided systematic supports for the accessibility of orphan drugs.

First, the implementation of compassionate drug use for rare diseases that aligns with China's national conditions is in effect. Compassionate drug use allows patients with rare diseases to use experimental drugs that have not yet been approved, including experimental drugs that have not entered a foreign market. According to the provisions of the Pharmaceutical Administration Law, drugs used for life-threatening diseases with no available and effective treatment currently, which may benefit from medical observation and comply with ethical principles, can be used for other patients with the same condition within the institution conducting clinical trials after review and informed consent. In June 2021, iptacopan for the treatment of Paroxysmal Nocturnal Hemoglobinuria (PNH) was successfully introduced and implemented at PUMCH, marking the pioneering journey of compassionate drug use in China.

Second, a market exclusivity period is granted for orphan drugs. China is actively exploring the implementation of a data protection system. In May 2022, the National Medical Products Administration issued a draft for public opinion on the revision of the *Implementation Regulations of the Pharmaceutical Administration Law of the People's Republic of China* (hereinafter referred to as the Draft for Public Opinion). Article 40 of the Draft for Public Opinion introduces 'data protection', expanding the scope of data protection beyond the current Article 34, which grants data protection of six years to producers or sellers of drugs with new chemical entities. The draft aims to establish a system for drug data protection for 'approved drugs', further advancing legislative efforts on drug data protection in China since 2002. In 2022, the *Implementation Regulations of the Pharmaceutical Administration Law (Draft for Public Opinion)* mentioned market exclusivity of up to 7 years for orphan drugs for the first time.

Thirdly, a pathway for the temporary importation of clinically urgent drugs that meet certain conditions is opened. In October 2018, the National Medical Products Administration, in collaboration with the National Health Commission, issued the *Announcement on Matters*

Related to the Review and Approval of Urgently Needed Overseas New Drugs for Clinical Use (Announcement No. 79 of 2018), establishing a dedicated pathway for the review and approval of urgently needed overseas new drugs for clinical use. Three lists of urgently needed overseas new drug varieties were selected and released, encouraging companies to apply. Among the 81 varieties in these three lists, over 50% were drugs for rare disease treatment. At present, 23 rare disease drugs have been approved for marketing through the special channel for overseas new drugs in urgent clinical need.

On June 29, 2022, the National Health Commission and the National Medical Products Administration jointly issued the *Work Plan for Temporary Importation of Clinically Urgent Drugs* and the *Work Plan for Temporary Importation of Iptacopan*, clarifying that a small quantity of urgently needed overseas marketed drugs, which are not registered for sale domestically, are not manufactured by domestic companies, or cannot be domestically produced in the short term, can be introduced into China through temporary importation. This approach better meets the clinical medication needs for rare diseases and other critical diseases. In August 2022, under the leadership of PUMCH, the first batch of imported drugs of Iptacopan for the treatment of refractory rare epilepsy entered China. The first prescription was issued on September 22, marking the formal establishment of the temporary importation pathway for urgently needed drugs, which innovated the mechanism with Chinese characteristics for orphan drug accessibility, paved the way for other orphan drugs, and stimulated drug development in related fields. On October 22, 2022, the first domestically produced generic Iptacopan by Yichang Renfu Pharmaceutical Co., Ltd. was launched, accelerating the process of domestic production of orphan drugs.

Fourth, we will strengthen the monitoring and guarantee of the production of medicines, including rare diseases drugs. In July 2022, the Ministry of Industry and Information Technology, the National Health Commission, the National Healthcare Security Administration and the National Medical Products Administration jointly issued the Notice on Strengthening the Monitoring of Production and Reserve of Shortage Medicines and Medicines Selected in the Centralized Purchase of Medicines by the Government, which established and improved the "Platform for Monitoring and Early Warning of Production and Supply of Shortage Medicines" . We should strengthen the dynamic monitoring and analysis of the production, circulation and stockpiling of key drugs, including drugs for rare diseases, improve the guarantee for the production scheduling and elements, and resolve the difficulties of production of enterprises on a "case-by-case" basis with regard to the drugs that are likely to be in short supply, so as to enhance the ability to ensure the supply of drugs for rare diseases.

Fifth, we will strongly support the industrialization of drugs for rare diseases. The Ministry of Industry and Information Technology, the National Development and Reform Commission and other departments implemented "14th Five-Year Plan for the Development of the Pharmaceutical Industry", aiming to strengthen policy synergies and strongly support the pharmaceutical industry to promote the industrialization of innovative products for the treatment of rare diseases. Through the existing funding channels, we will beef up support for projects, recommend the upstream and downstream industry chain enterprises and scientific research units to strengthen collaboration, support the establishment of public platforms for the production of drugs for rare diseases, carry out research on key technologies, strengthen the points of weakness of the industry chain, and effectively improve the industrialization of drugs for rare diseases.

V. Steady Progress of the Social Security System for Rare Diseases

The Chinese government attaches importance to social security for rare diseases, not only by means of basic medical insurance, social insurance, social welfare and social assistance led by government, but also via promotion of diverse social forces including philanthropy and commercial insurance facilitated by government. In recent years, social security has registered rapid progresses, and the reform and exploration of social security for rare diseases call for stronger courage and commitment.

1. Medical insurance for rare diseases

(1) Systems and policies

On February 25, 2020, the CPC Central Committee and the State Council issued the *Opinions on Deepening the Reform of Medical insurance System*, calling for exploring the guarantee mechanism for medications of rare diseases. In January 2021, the National Healthcare Security Administration and the Ministry of Finance jointly issued the

Opinions on Establishing Management System of a List of Medical Insurance Benefits, further clarifying the scope of basic medical insurance and distinguishing between the coverage of basic medical insurance and commercial health insurance.

In October 2021, the General Office of the State Council issued the *Opinions on Improving the Medical Insurance and Assistance System for Severe and Rare Diseases*, calling for the exploration of a guarantee mechanism for orphan drugs based on the economic and social development level and the capacity of all parties involved through the integration of medical insurance, social assistance, charitable support, and other resources to implement comprehensive support. Medical insurance authorities have resolutely implemented the decisions of the State Council of the CPC Central Committee and carefully studied approaches to strengthen medical insurance for patients with rare diseases, So far, a unified and synergic medical insurance system for urban and rural residents has been established, integrating basic medical insurance, medical insurance for patients with critical illnesses, and medical assistance.

First, medical insurance benefits have been steadily improved. At present, the in-patient reimbursement ratios for employees and residents (urban and rural) are 80% and 70% respectively. Critical illness insurance for urban and rural residents has been comprehensively implemented. In 2019, the deductible for critical illness insurance was reduced to half of the per capita disposable income of the previous year, and the reimbursement ratio for medical expenses increased to 60%; in addition, preferential reimbursement policy has been introduced for the impoverished population.

Second, eligible drugs for rare diseases will be gradually covered by the basic medical insurance system. In accordance with the *Interim Measures on the Drug Administration of Basic Medical Insurance*, the reimbursed drug list will be reviewed every year, which means that more eligible drugs that have completed application, expert review, market access negotiation, and other compulsory procedures will be reimbursed by medical insurance. For the 121 diseases included in the list of the first batch of rare diseases, most of the medicines and medical services for these diseases have been covered by the medical insurance system. To address the actual clinical medication needs of patients with rare diseases, the *2022 National Basic Medical Insurance, Work-related Injury Insurance, and Maternity Insurance Drug List Adjustment Plan* provides further preferential reimbursement towards special populations such as patients with rare diseases, and the application for orphan drugs is not subject to the 5-year approval restriction. The Drug Catalogue of National Basic Medical Insurance, Work Injury Insurance and Maternity Insurance (2022) includes more than 50 medicines for rare diseases. covering 27 rare diseases, including drugs for the treatment of idiopathic pulmonary hypertension (IPAH), C-type Niemann Pick's disease, early-onset Parkinson's disease (EOPD), idiopathic pulmonary fibrosis (IPS), Huntington's disease (HD) and other diseases. In 2021, the cost of Nusinersen Sodium Injection for the treatment of Spinal Muscular Atrophy (SMA) decreased from nearly CNY 700,000 per injection to approximately CNY 33,000, a reduction of over 95%. A total of 26 rare disease medicines have been included in the list of medicines covered by the medical-insurance system through negotiation, with an average price reduction of more than 50%.

Third, medical assistance mechanism has been strengthened for those most in need. With regard to patients with rare diseases who are low-income-insurance recipients, persons in special hardship, or those who have returned to poverty, the government will coordinate efforts to increase outpatient and inpatient assistance, with the proportion of eligible medical expenses covered by the annual assistance limit being approximately 70 per cent, and the annual assistance limit reaching 30,000 to 50,000 yuan. Local governments also take into account their medical assistance funds and the needs of the needy, and appropriately expand the scope of assistance recipients by promptly including families of patients with rare diseases who have incurred high medical expenses. Through the three-tier system of basic medical insurance, major disease insurance and medical assistance, the actual reimbursement ratio of medical expenses for the rural low-income population has reached about 80 per cent. In April 2021, the National Healthcare Security Administration and seven other ministries issued the *Implementation Opinions on Consolidating and Expanding the Achievements of Healthcare Security in Poverty Alleviation and Effectively Linking with the Rural Revitalization Strategy*. On the basis of the comprehensive implementation of inclusive policies for critical illness insurance, this initiative provides enhanced support for people in dire poverty, subsistence allowance recipients, and those who have returned or been reduced to poverty, including a 50% reduction in the deductible, a 5 percentage point increase in the reimbursement rate, and a gradual removal of the preferential reimbursement for the limit line.

(2) Measures to reduce costs

Since 2018, the medical insurance authority and relevant departments have carried out centralized volume-based procurement (VBP) of generic drugs that have successfully passed consistency evaluation of quality and efficacy with multiple competitors. Orphan drugs including Ambrisentan have been included in the centralized procurement scheme, with bidding price down to 20 yuan per tablet from 100 yuan. Currently, VBP has been rolled out nationwide and has become a regular work. Gradually, more medicines will be included in centralized volume purchase, so as to eliminate the inflated prices of medicines.

(3) Local pilots and experience

Local governments have actively explored the path of medical insurance for rare diseases, and have alleviated the burden of high medical costs on patients with special rare diseases in their regions by exploring a sound multi-tier medical insurance system. They have explored their own distinctive path and accumulated valuable experience. These provinces have launched pilot medical and social security systems for rare diseases, taking into account local patients as well as financial and medical insurance fund affordability. Various security models of rare diseases with local characteristics have been established. In short, The multi-tier social security system, which is evolving and improving rapidly, and is now providing a strong shelter for patients with rare diseases to live a dignified and promising life.

2. Social security for rare diseases

Social security has always been the core concern of the prevention and treatment of rare diseases; medical insurance for rare diseases has been the focus of attention from of the whole society. Up to now, China has preliminarily established a complete legal system of social security for rare diseases, mainly including the *Constitution of the People's Republic of China, the Education Law of the People's Republic of China,* the *Labor Law of the People's Republic of China,* the *Social Insurance Law of the People's Republic of China,* the *Charity Law of the People's Republic of China,* the *Interim Measures for Social Assistance,* etc. At the same time, clear arrangements have been made for social insurance, social assistance, social welfare, and other aspects of social security for rare diseases in China. Nevertheless, due to the current level of economic and social development in China, social security for rare diseases in

China is still in its initial stage. Social security supports for rare diseases are mostly integrated in the general social security scheme for all the Chinese population. A relatively independent, specialized and tailored social security scheme for rare diseases is yet to be designed.

(1) Strengthened social assistance

Social assistance for vulnerable groups with low or no income, including patients living with rare diseases, has always been an important government agenda. Social assistance capacity of the Chinese government is constantly improving, so is the level of social assistance. Local departments of civil affairs have provided subsistence allowances for eligible patients with rare diseases, as well as relief and support and temporary assistance for people in dire poverty in a timely manner. To increase assistance for children with genetic metabolic diseases, the Department of Maternal and Child Health of the National Health Commission (former National Health and Family Planning Commission) has actively joined hands with organizations such as the March of Dimes Birth Defects Foundation of China to launch and implement birth defects relief programs since 2016; more than 20 rare diseases such as methylmalonic aciduria and phenylketonuria were included in the *List of the First Batch of Rare Diseases*. As of July 2020,, more than 3,100 children with rare diseases have received assistance allowances, and over 29 million yuan has been allocated for the purpose of medical insurance and assistance. The project has continuously expanded the scope of medical assistance for children with rare diseases, which now covers a wide range of rare diseases, including genetic and metabolic, neurological, cardiovascular, digestive, dermatological, urological, ophthalmological, immunological and hematological, as well as endocrine and metabolic disorders, thus improving medical insurance and assistance for children living with rare diseases and effectively reducing the financial and psychological burden for families of those children.

(2) Expanded coverage of social insurance

Our social insurance efforts have provided, through legislative means, an increasing number of social insurance benefits for our people, including those with rare diseases. The *Law of the People's Republic of China on Social Insurance* enacted in 2010, has laid a legal foundation for the institutional arrangements and systematic operations of the social insurance system in China. China has achieved full coverage of social insurance, 1.345 billion people are covered by basic medical insurance nationwide, with 362 million in medical insurance for urban employees and 983 million in medical insurance for residents. 1.05 billion people are covered by basic old-age insurance nationwide. Specifically, employees with rare diseases who are enrolled in the basic old-age insurance system are entitled to basic old-age insurance benefits when they meet requirements for entitlement; other patients with rare diseases may choose to get enrolled in the basic old-age insurance for employees of enterprises or the basic old-age insurance for urban and rural residents in accordance with their realities, so that they are entitled to the corresponding old-age insurance benefits when they meet the requirements for entitlement. Through the work injury insurance and unemployment insurance, China has set up a work injury and unemployment relief system with Chinese characteristics for workers injured at work and the unemployed, including those with rare diseases.

(3) Encouraged social participation

In 2016, China published and implemented the Charity Law of the Peoples Republic of China, which provides new guarantee and impetus for social charity forces in China to contribute to social security for rare diseases. The first charitable foundation for rare disease in China is Rare Disease Relief Public Welfare Fund launched by China Charity Federation on December 23, 2009. According to preliminary statistics, as of 2015, there were more than 20 rare disease charity funds in China, and this number has continued to increase in recent years.

In December 2021, the Rare Disease Alliance of China and the China Red Cross Foundation jointly initiated the "Rare Disease Co-funding Fund", dedicated not only to providing assistance to patients with rare diseases and spreading knowledge about rare diseases but also to supporting projects related to rare disease physician training, research, and technological development in the public interest. In addition to providing assistance as private-sector players, some of the rare disease public welfare funds also participated in the reform of the medical and social security system for rare diseases and were also included in the social security mechanism of local govemments'co-payment mechanism for rare diseases. In the meantime, some patient organizations have also gradually developed and gained influence and organizational capacity, such as Beijing Oriental Rain ALS Care Center (BORACC), which focuses on ALS, and Beijing Illness Challenge Foundation, a comprehensive charity organization that fosters rare disease community groups. As of September 2019, there were more than 80 rare disease non-profit organizations in China.

(4) Highlight the supplementary role of commercial insurance

Social security for rare diseases requires more participation from various sectors of society. In recent years, local governments have successively launched people-oriented commercial medical insurances that co-work with basic medical insurance, and some of these insurances have tried to include a small number of rare disease drugs. For example, in Shandong Province, most "Hui Min Bao" products have included drugs for rare diseases. In April 2021, Shanghai released "Hu Hui Bao," which includes three orphan drugs and five high-value drugs in its specific high-cost drug list, with a maximum coverage of up to 1 million yuan. According to data provided by the China Banking and Insurance Regulatory Commission, more than 200 critical illness insurance products have included certain rare diseases. In terms of medical insurance, most commercial medical insurance products cover medical expenses for patients with rare diseases, providing financial guarantee for those with critical illnesses. The aforementioned demonstrates the supplementary role of insurance beyond the scope of basic medical insurance, which not only helps the government alleviate the pressure of medical insurance expenditure and reduce the overall treatment costs for patients with rare diseases but also offers these patients the opportunity for equitable treatment within its capabilities.

VI. Active Participation in International Cooperation of Rare Diseases Prevention and Treatment

China has maintained close contact and communication with other countries in the world in capacity building of rare disease prevention and management. While learning from the advanced management experience from foreign countries, China also shares its practices and experience while working with the rest of the world for continuous progresses in the prevention and treatment of rare diseases. Since 2014, China has been sending delegates to participate in the first and second sessions of the UN Committee of NGOs on Rare Diseases to learn from the experience of other countries, communicate policies related to rare diseases in China, and share our achievements. Many universities and medical institutions in China have actively cooperated with international organizations in researches on rare diseases, making a series of significant progress. In addition, a number of social organizations in China have actively cooperated with international organizations in holding academic conferences on rare diseases as well as launching education campaigns and patient care programs, which have greatly promoted social awareness of rare diseases in China.

The China Conference on Rare Diseases was held in October 2022. Representatives from organizations such as the World Health Organization (WHO) in China, the International Alliance of Patients' Organizations for Rare Diseases (IAPO), and the United Nations NGO Committee for Rare Diseases, highly commended China's approach of defining rare diseases in the form of a catalog, and acknowledged the significant achievements made in exploring the path with Chinese characteristics for rare disease diagnosis, treatment, and guarantee.

On July 15, 2023, the "First International Medical Genomics Summit" was successfully held in Beijing. This conference was jointly organized by the China Alliance for Rare Diseases / Beijing Society of Rare Disease Clinical Care and Accessibility and the Beijing Ruiyang Bohui Charity Foundation. The summit, with the focus on the latest technological developments of whole genome sequencing (WGS) both domestically and internationally. The event served as a platform to showcase domestic academic accomplishments and engage in discussions surrounding pertinent industry standards. The overarching objective was to leverage China's expertise in genomics to contribute to its global advancement.

Conclusion

Health is the enduring pursuit of mankind, and we are unwavering in our commitment to safeguarding the rights related to the health of patients living with rare diseases. This endeavor holds great significance in upholding the right to health for the Chinese population. President Xi Jinping has emphasized that national prosperity is inseparable from the well-being of its citizens, making the strengthening of rare disease prevention and treatment a vital task in advancing the creation of a Healthy China. Furthermore, it is an essential requirement for the holistic development of a moderately prosperous society, aligning perfectly with the sentiments of the public and the decisions and directives of the CPC Central Committee and the State Council. Departments involved have actively implemented the principles set forth by the CPC Central Committee and the State Council, successively issuing policies for the prevention, treatment, and guarantee of rare diseases. Thanks to years of unremitting efforts, remarkable progresses have been achieved in the formulation of policies and systems, clinical diagnosis and treatment, drug supply mechanism, social security system, major scientific research breakthroughs, international cooperation and exchanges. As a result, an increasing number of patients afflicted with rare diseases have gained access to diagnosis, treatment, and comprehensive care.

Nowadays, rare disease prevention and treatment has gone through a rapid development period and has entered a period of adjustment and improvement. Looking forward, further improving the top-level design and legislations for social security policy, innovating the guarantee framework for orphan drugs, strengthening support for R&D of diagnostic and treatment technologies and drugs, ensuring the stable supply of orphan drugs, and introducing more supportive policies will be the priorities for the prevention and treatment of rare diseases in China.

The Party and the State have proactively explored and practiced the pathway of rare disease diagnosis, treatment, and guarantee. Governments at all levels will continue to uphold a strong sense of responsibility and urgency, striving to comprehensively ensure people's health for the full-life cycle, and promoting the overall development of medical and health services. All sectors of society will continue to collaborate in an ongoing effort to improve the "Chinese model" of rare disease diagnosis, treatment, and security system, realizing the vision where patients with rare diseases can receive timely diagnosis and treatment under effective management, while ensuring that orphan drugs are both accessible and affordable for patients grappling with rare diseases.